My Story

My Story

"A Bump on the Road"

Edwin G. Camargo

iUniverse, Inc.
New York   Lincoln   Shanghai

My Story
"A Bump on the Road"

iUniverse books may be ordered through booksellers or by contacting:

iUniverse
2021 Pine Lake Road, Suite 100
Lincoln, NE 68512
www.iuniverse.com
1-800-Authors (1-800-288-4677)

ISBN-13: 978-0-595-39290-2 (pbk)
ISBN-13: 978-0-595-83683-3 (ebk)
ISBN-10: 0-595-39290-3 (pbk)
ISBN-10: 0-595-83683-6 (ebk)

Printed in the United States of America

Contents

Life

My short journey through life has taught me that life is hard. It has no empty roads but a lot of bumps and turns. Trust me when I say that I am in the worst roller coaster imaginable. I have made all the wrong turns and I have learned that the only way to take control is to learn from my actions. I was in a dark…very dark place once. My back was against the wall, and I wished that I was dead at one point. Death seemed like the only solution but now I am glad that I am still here walking towards the moon and reaching for the stars.

A new Edwin emerged from the darkness. An Edwin that one day will make a name for himself. The lessons that I have learned have turn me into a better man; into someone who understands why he is here and an individual who lives life like there is no tomorrow. I am now a new man who lives life with a smile on his face. I am a man who helps others and most importantly I'm someone that desires a new life.

Slow and steady wins the race. Take your time, enjoy every second because time doesn't forgive anyone and it doesn't walk backwards. Take advantage of every opportunity and increase your odds. Take a chance and roll the dice hoping to turn the odds around. Our actions define who we are. We have the power to choose our path, our lifestyle and our destiny.

Being only 22 years of age you might think that I am not the one to be talking about life but please let me tell you my story

Edwin

My name is Edwin, but for most of my family I am Geovanny, my middle name. My last name is really not important, but if you're like me, and you must know it is Camargo. I was born in Los Angeles, California. It was on March 31, 1983 when my eyes saw light for the first time. March 31st was a warm, blooming spring Sunday; at least that is what my mom says. My mom is from a small calm town in El Salvador called Cojutepeque and my dad is from Chilpancingo, Mexico. Chilpancingo is a quiet, violence free town two hours away from Acapulco. Both my parents grew up in a farm environment away from the city. They are both very smart but unfortunately neither have a high school diploma. My dad used to be in the Mexican army.

I am the oldest of three. I have two brothers, Wilbert is two years younger than me, and Elmer is eleven years younger than me.

Unfortunately I have no sisters. All that I am stuck with is just two mischievous brothers that whine like little girls sometimes. Just a few weeks after my birth my parents moved to Chilpancingo, Guerrero in Mexico. Like I mentioned Chilpancingo is a small, quiet town located just a few miles south of Acapulco. It was there where my childhood began. I attended kindergarten and first grade of elementary school in Chilpancingo. As a matter of fact, I attended the same elementary school where my aunt teaches sixth grade. My brother Wilbert was born in Chilpancingo. In 1990 my parents decided to migrate back to the United States. We settled in Anaheim, California. However, a few weeks later we moved to Orange County; also in California. In 1994, my brother Elmer was born.

My parents worked very hard to provide me and my brother with the best. My parents worked at a local senior citizen living complex called Park Plaza. My dad is the chef and my mom the dinning room supervisor. For a short time I too worked at Park Plaza. I worked in the front desk, but unlike my parents I was only there for about 4 months, and I only worked on Sundays.

After many years of shyness, quietness, out-sider ness, and hard work I graduated in the year of 2001. I graduated from Orange High School. Then I attend Cal State Fullerton University. Now that you know a bit about myself let me tell you about my short journey in life.

My Early Years

Like most kids, growing up was about having fun and discovering new things. As a young kid I always had a smile on my face, well that is what my mom says. I don't remember much about my childhood. However, I do remember most of my mischievous acts. For example, I do remember, one time when my grandmother was cooking beans in a big pot. What happened next you won't believe! But when she was not looking I threw rocks inside the pot. Like every one, I didn't get away with it. I was punished for a couple of days. As a small child I was not the friend type. What I mean is that I did not have many friends. As a matter of fact I only remember having one friend, Veronica Guzman, my neighbor. Veronica and I had many adventures growing up. I remember that once, we threw her mom's expensive cream all over our bodies. That day we went into her house regular kids and we came out looking like two miniature clowns. Her mom's angry face still haunts me to this day. Everybody else who I played with was family. My cousins lived nearby. While I was in Chilpancingo I grew up in a spacious house. It had four bedrooms, two bathrooms; the house also had a big kitchen and a rose filled garden in the front. The house also had walk in closets, which I used as a hiding place when I did something bad. My grandmother's house was in the same plantation and only a shout away if I ever needed her protection. I don't remember much of my early years but my grandma says that I spend a lot of time hiding from my mom in her house, I guess I had done something wrong and I new I was going to get it, so I hid.

However, when we moved back to the states we lived in a small I bedroom apartment. I was very sad because I had lost my best friend and my cousins. So, with my brother growing up I began to play more frequent with him. After a couple of weeks of sadness my parents bought me and my brother the hottest game, Nintendo. Soon the afternoons became all about who could pass the most levels in Super Mario 3, with my brother's help I was able to pass every level. By that point marbles were "in" and I began to forget about the Nintendo and began to focus on my shooting skills. For the next couple of years it was all about playing for keeps and making my marble collection grow. Now I am soon to be 21 and fun is one of the few things that inspire me to get up every morning.

At only 20 years of age I have learned that life is filled with obstacles. However, no matter how many times I have to prove to my self that I can do it. Fun is never too far behind. Not even 21 yet, the hardest obstacle I have faced is to live with multiple sclerosis. Living with M.S., multiple sclerosis, is not easy. I've had to deal with this disorder every long day of my life for the past year and a half. Living with M.S. is a violent fight that I have to put up with every day; a fight that scares me to death because I know what the outcome may be. The symptoms are not pretty, and make every day life very difficult. I have to deal with weakness, hypersensitivity, numbness, stiffness. I may be dealing with blindness, and not being able to maintain proper balance. These are some of the problems that I face every day.

Life in general is surprisingly difficult. The harder you work; the happier you are. "Why?" you ask. Because the more you work the more success you have and success is the road to happiness. Life is like an empty highway. The faster you get to your final destination; the happier you are. In life, your final destination is retirement with wealth and success. I had everything set, an empty road, a fast car and a brilliant mind to reach retirement the quickest way possible. Unfortunately, M.S. is a bump, a big bump, on the road that has altered my road to success.

Who Am I?

Growing up in the Hispanic culture was not a smooth ride. My parents have always pressure me into being the best that I can be. As a child, that always meant attending school, and studying every single night. Everyday after school I had to run home because my mom had to go to work and I needed to take care of the house. Being the oldest of three, I was to set the prime example for my brothers. Like everyone, school was a challenge. Especially at first, because I knew absolutely no English when I came back from Mexico. Fortunately, I picked up the language little by little. My teachers have always told me that I have an intelligent mind. In school, I was the quiet one in the back. I was the outsider, who only wanted to work by himself. I was the shy one, who did not want to talk. An intelligent mind is a great weapon to have when conquering education. Believe it or not I have never studied for a test or quiz in my life. It was plain and simple for me. All that I had to do was to attend class and pay attention every day. When it came test time: the test answered itself. I have never failed any important test, and I have never receive a grade lower than an 85%. I consider myself a good test taker. However, being able to take tests, and answer questions is not the only solution to the problems we face every day.

Knowledge is the only key to success. There is no one in this world that will hand you this key. You must earn this key by experiencing the game of life. A game of trial and error that is difficult to beat. Education is probably the best alliance against this twisted game.

Education starts the very first day we see the light. It is our parents who take care of us. They are our first teachers, and best friend. They teach us to eat, talk, walk, and how to defend ourselves without using violence. Our parents are the only teachers that stand by our side every step of the way.

Nobody is perfect. We all have our weaknesses and strengths. For me math is one of my strengths. I like figuring out the solution to problems that will help me out in life.

Furthermore, I love the thrill of solving math problems. I have always loved history, another of my strong points. History teaches us about the mistakes other people have made in the past and hopefully that will prevent me from making the same mistakes in my future. Science will always be there, so I have always tried to understand it as much as possible. In high school science became a difficult challenge to overcome.

Sports have always been difficult for me. Other than basketball, physical activities are a weakness, a weakness that I have struggle with most of my childhood life. Being the last one to be picked makes you feel like you're not wanted. It hurts emotionally and can damage your ego. All that you can do is to try your best, and forget about what others think. After being diagnose with M.S. I will probably never achieve the thought of being more athletic. I have always been shy. Being the shy one made talking to people a weakness. Being the shy one in the class also made presentations very difficult. I have never felt passionate about art. I can't draw and I can't paint. Art is the weakness that I wish would just disappear. Grammar is another of my weaknesses. I love to write, whether it was essays, poetry, and everything else in between. My teachers have always liked my writing: it is my grammar that they dislike.

Knowledge being the key to success is not only found through education but through experience as well.

My Big Break

Education has always been a priority in life, and I believe that is why I loved school. My love for school was so great that I was one of the few students to be awarded the perfect attendance award every year in high school. As a matter of fact, I only remember missing a total of 5 days from school my entire life. I was also a recipient of the principle's honor roll every year for my outstanding grade point average always being higher than a 3.5.

Unfortunately, the great success that I was having in school was not enough for me. My sophomore year of high school I decided that I wanted to explore the real world. So, I enlisted in a course offered by the Regional Opportunity Program. I registered in a banking and finance course. My teacher was Mrs. Backstrom; she had many years of experience, and had managed banks for many years as well. I learned basic policies and to use the ten key. I was one of the quickest using the ten key; I was typing at a speed of almost 100 numbers per minute (above average). I felt in love with this class and that's when I knew what I wanted to study in college. This course offered me the opportunity to have an internship with Bank of America. I didn't have to think it twice. I immediately accepted it. For the following 3 months I went to a Bank of America located inside Main Place, a mall in Orange. I learned simple tasks, and I learned how to assist customers. Knowing that banks only hire persons of 18 years of age or older. At only 16 and a half I applied for a position with Bank of America. During my internship I had demonstrated my skills and love for the job. Just a few days after applying I received a call from Miss Hector, one of the recruiters.

Miss Hector asked me to go in for an interview. She told me the date and time, and just an hour later I told my dad. With a big smile, and filled with joy we began to arrange how he was to take me to the interview. Since I didn't have a car, my dad had no problem taking me. When the time arrived to prove myself I was very nervous and it was impossible for Ms. Hector not to notice. My palms were sweaty and I felt like I was being cooked in an oven. To make it worse I was shaking like maracas. The first thing she said was, "relax I am only going to ask you a couple questions". It was all a big lie. The intense interview lasted about an hour. Even though, it took an hour to get an answer, she asked me to come back in a few days for testing. Two days later I returned for testing.

I was not the only one there. There were probably six of us. The way I saw it, they were my competition. After three hours of trick questions, it was time for the results. One by one we were taken to a back office, and told our scores. I had a perfect score, and Miss Hector asked me to set up an interview with the branch manager of where I wanted to work. So I called the manager. Unfortunately, he was on vacation and I had to interview with the assisting manager. Her name was Miss Blanco. She was a mean looking woman, whose first question was, "how old are you?" I told her I was 16 soon to turn 17. The mean expression on her face changed and appeared to be surprised. Then she asked, "What grade are you in?" I answered, "10". After half an hour she told me I had the job, and this became one of the happiest times of my life. I became the youngest person to work for Bank of America or any other bank.

I had to attend a two week training session before starting. That became trouble because the training classes started at 1 o'clock in the afternoon. Since I had extra class credits I was able to move my class schedule around so that I would be able to leave by 12:15 noon. The problem was that the training classes were located in another city. Since I did not have a car or a driver's license I had to run to the bus stop because in order for me to make the training I had to get on the 12:30 bus. The nearest bus stop was approximately 1.5 miles away so I really had to hurry. I remember that I did miss the bus once and I had to wait for the next bus. Luckily the trainer did not get mad at me for arriving almost an hour late.

Like everyone, I began at the bottom. Being a teller was not easy. I had a lot of responsibilities. The most important was to balance my box every night. It didn't take long to fit in. My great attitude made it a lot easier. All of my co-workers thought I was about 21. Just about a year after working, the merchant teller position opened. The manager offered me the position, and I accepted it. That night I told my parents and filled with joy they took us, my brothers and I, out for dinner. The new position came along with more responsibilities. The most important was balancing the vault and the large amount in my new box every night. It took me about 3 weeks to understand all of my responsibilities. Through out this time I was awarded many certificates for my hard work, integrity, and my teamwork. But just after a few months I was awarded one of the most precious awards. I was awarded the Leadership Cup Award. After a year of working the merchant window I was promoted to teller coach. Now with bigger pay and better benefits I was responsible for training new employees. It felt great to be on top of the world.

Attending school and working was not easy. Even though, I had a great paying job my main priority was school. It is because of that, that I was working part time. As a sophomore in high school I was able to put aside my work and focus on school every morning. It was difficult at first, but I was still able to maintain my good grades. My life was becoming a great success at such a young age. I was very happy with my life. I had a great paying job, and success in school. The most important was having proud parents.

My junior year was the most difficult for me. That year I was taking physics, pre-calculus, and chemistry. Even though it became harder to maintain good grades, I was able to work 5 days of the week. Half way through the school year I bought my first car. For the remainder of the year I drove an old, cherry red, 1990 Chrysler Lebaron that needed new paint.

I was soon to turn 18 when I met Jessica. It was a busy Thursday when I assisted her for the first time. For the next three weeks I assisted her every Thursday. On the following Thursday, filled with butterflies in my stomach, I asked her out. She turned cherry red. Little did I know that the customer in the next window was her mother. It took her a few minutes but she accepted my offer. Since it was busy, I asked her for her phone number. Later that night I called her and apologized for embarrassing her in front of her mother. Anyways, for the next year my relationship with her grew bigger and bigger by the day. Jessica had a beautiful white smile and soft curly hair. She was outgoing, and wild. Everyday was filled with joy, understanding, and happiness. Jessica was Honduran and had been living in the U.S for the last three months. She spoke fairly well English, but that was no problem since I am bilingual. Like most guys, my first love made me walk on air, and she became number one. Jessica was my date to prom. I rented a midnight blue limousine just for the two of us. That clear sky, cold night I became a man.

Aside from my personal life, in high school, I was able to join the National Honors' Society and graduate in the top 5% of my class. I graduated the warm summer of 2001. After high school, I declined a scholarship to Washington State University because I did not want to move away from my family. Instead I attended Cal State University Fullerton. I was studying finance and business administration. I was attending school full time. I took classes in the morning, worked 10am-7pm, and also took classes at night. College was different. Having the opportunity to schedule your own class time was difficult for me. There were so many classes to choose from, and I wanted them all. The classes were big, and learning became self-initiated. If I wanted to pass the class I was responsible for learning the subject by my self. The professor's, in my mind, did not do much teaching. Unlike high school where I had to pay attention in class to pass the subject; in college I had to read books over and over again. I did not like it one bit.

After my first year in college my relationship ended with Jessica. After several months of joy and understanding; my relationship with Jessica came to an end. Our relationship had lasted about a year. The reason why we broke up was that we just stopped understanding ourselves. We were not communicating like we used to, and frankly our feelings had changed. Although it was a mutual breakup I was in pain. It hurt and up to this day I still don't understand why? My mom never did like Jessica, so she was really happy when it was all over.

Soon after ending my relationship with Jessica I decided that it was time for a change. I bought a new car, and began searching for a new job. Cruising in a brand new, silver cougar I began seeking new employment.

My Luck

I don't like to attend church, and to be honest with you I am not much of a believer. It was a cold and rainy Sunday. My mom had me clinched by the ear and forced me to take her to church. My plans were just to drop her off but when we arrived there, I saw an angel entering church and that was when I decided to enter as well. We sat on the row behind her, and across from her. It was only a couple of months after breaking up with Jessica when I was beginning to fall in love again. I did not talk with her that cold Sunday, but for the next several Sundays I invited her out for coffee, tea, an ice cream, and even for a cup of juice. Unfortunately, her answer was always no.

I had been searching for a job for some time now. When I found the perfect place, I applied for a Member Service Representative position with the Orange County Teacher's Federal Credit Union, OCTFCU. It only took a few days before I went in for an interview. My interviewer's name was Michelle. She had recently been hired and I was her first recruit. She was very friendly and it only took the following day before I knew I was hired. I gave my two-week notice to B of A, but unhappy with my decision they tried to pursue me by offering me better pay. Unfortunately, for Bank of America, OCTFCU had offered me a better package. Unhappy, with my decision, B of A let me go just a week later. For me, that meant that I had a little over a week to start at my new job.

I decided that I was going to take a short vacation. The next day I went to school and told my teachers of what I was planning on doing. I asked my teachers for the work that I would be missing. Fortunately, none of them opposed. That Sunday I gave that shiny angel my number, and told her to give me a call if she was interested. That day I learned that her name was Magda. The following day I was on a plane to Acapulco, Mexico. I spend my time there relaxing under the hot sun. My stay in Acapulco flew right by me. I didn't want to return home, but I knew I had to.

I arrived home on a Sunday. The next day I would be starting at my new job. Before talking about my new job I want to share with you what happened on the Sunday evening I returned home.

It was about 3 o'clock in the afternoon when I arrived home. First thing I did was check my cell phone for missed calls and messages. At that very moment my cell phone rang. It was very odd since no one knew that I had returned. It was Magda, but instead of telling me who she was she told me her name was Mariela. She was playing me a prank; to see how I would respond. Knowing it had to be Magda I played along. I was very excited about having a girl looking for me. She began to tell me how we had met; since I had no idea were or how. I told her that I didn't remember her, and asked her to describe herself. She told me she was about my height (about 5"11), dark blonde hair, and blue eyes. I continued to play along by saying. "Yes I remember you. We met at that place." Then she told me how we had met at Nordstrom, a store at the mall. Her lying prank continued for two more days. When she finally confessed I told her that after a prank like that I deserved a date. The following Saturday I got my date. We went to the mall where I asked her to show me where I met Mariela. We then enjoyed a delicious cup of coffee. It was there were I learned that she was 24 years old, but did not look a day pass 20. She had beautiful deep, mysterious brown eyes, a big white smile, about 5 feet 4 inches tall, thin, sexy, and a great set of wheel to carry her anywhere.

I continued to see Magda. But my new job soon became a little more important. I was very happy with my new job. I was now earning about $5,000 more per year and had fewer responsibilities. My new environment felt great. It felt like Disneyland. I was now working for the happiest and friendliest people on earth. The hardest part of my new job was referring to customers as Members. My main priority was to provide Members with world-class service. My fun loving life there didn't last long. Just a few days after starting there I began to feel numbness in my right hand. At first I did not worry much, but soon after the numbness began to walk to my elbow. My luck was changing. After having found the women of my dreams and a good job, my luck was unexpectedly changing.

My Darkest Hour

The following weekend I saw my doctor. Dr. Bader ordered blood tests. He also told me that he believed I was dealing with Carpal Tunnel Syndrome. By Monday, my right foot began to feel numb. That afternoon I called Dr. Bader and asked him for the results of the lab work. He told me that the results were normal, and I began to tell him what I was feeling. He told me that he wanted to see me, and I scheduled an appointment for the following Monday. The following days my situation got worse. I began to feel a tingly sensation all over my body. I also began to feel stiffness in my right hand. By Saturday I began to loose control of my right hand, and began to feel weak. I began to feel like a dependent kid again. My parents had gotten worried and that Sunday they took me to the emergency room.

Unfortunately, my new health benefits had not been activated yet. I needed to have been working with OCTFCU for three months before receiving benefit of the company paid PPO Plan. Luckily for me, I was able to maintain my health benefits through COBRA. I paid a $200 monthly premium.

Anyways, the doctor in the emergency room had no answer on what I had. He ordered MRIs and arranged for me to see a neurologist. My appointment with the neurologist was set up for Tuesday. I did something that I had never done before in my life. I called in sick on Monday and Tuesday. That Tuesday I got to see Dr. Susan Skinner, the neurologist, but by then I had become weaker and number. Dr. Skinner was the director of the neurological department at Kaiser Permanente. I liked her and I felt comfortable with her. Dr. Skinner told me that I could be suffering from transverse mylitis. I asked her what that was. She told me that it was the starting stage of multiple sclerosis. She explained briefly that it was a condition when your nervous system does not work properly and your cells begin to kill each other. Not really understanding, I said okay and knotted my head. She needed to make sure, so she ordered a spinal tap. A spinal tap is when they insert a fine needle into your spinal cord to retrieve spinal fluid. She was going to precede this operation and scheduled the procedure for the following day. That same day I asked my dad to take me to the credit union. Since I had just started I had no right to any time off beside sick days. I knew that it was going to take time to recuperate. I saw myself forced to resign. That Tuesday was one of the worst days of my life. I had never quit before, so saying goodbye to my new friends was very difficult and emotional for me. Human recourses asked me to re-apply once I was ready. That same night I did research on what multiple sclerosis was. Well I had my brother do it but you get the idea. I learned that almost 65% of all cases are in woman. Also that it is more common in older people. On Wednesday I had a better idea of what I was dealing with. I was also terrified of what I had to go through later that day. A spinal tap is one of the most painful procedures that are practiced in the doctor's office. Friends and family members were telling me that it hurts a lot, maybe more than a broken bone. I only got scared more than what I already was. By the time I had the spinal tap done my body was so numb it was hard to walk. I felt so stiff that I didn't feel a thing. For a second, I thought that Dr. Skinner had not begin the procedure, but when I asked her she told me that they were almost done and not to move. Dr. Skinner told me that I also needed to have blood drawn. When it was all over, she called my parents, who had been waiting impatiently in the waiting room, to join me and told us that it was going to take a few days for the results to come in.

With my condition the way it was. I stopped attending class for about a week. With my condition not improving I was not able to attend school, and not being able to do many simple tasks. It was a decision that I had to make, and I stopped worrying about attending school.

While I waited for the results I learned that I had lost almost 75% of my strength. I also had to begin using my left hand because my right hand was not only stiff, but unmovable as well. My hand looked useless. I couldn't move it and it felt dead. It is in this close position with all my fingers cuddled up almost making an open fist. It looks like it is just hanging from my wrist. I can't open it and I can't even hold a pen or pencil. Since I am right handed the right side of my body was affected more. Depending on my parents for help was something that I disliked, so I refused almost every act of help. I have such a big ego that I never asked anyone for help. I began to believe that if I was not able do something today maybe tomorrow I'll have better luck. On Monday morning I received a call from my new doctor. Dr. Skinner asked us, my parents and me, to go in and see her. That afternoon we went in for the results.

By that afternoon I had gotten worse. Not only was I numb, weak, but by now my skin was hypersensitive. What I mean by hypersensitive is that my skin felt like the day after a burn. The slightest touch would sting. So, I began to use the least amount of clothes as possible.

It was July 20th in the year 2002, and the news I received that day scarred me for life. Dr. Skinner sat us down. She began to explain that I was dealing with a rare condition usually found in older individuals. At only 19 years of age I was told that I had multiple sclerosis. It felt really bad inside. It hurt. I felt my dreams shatter.

Like every parent, my parents could not believe it nor accept my condition. My mom with tears in her eyes asked Dr. Skinner to re-test me. She did, but no good news resulted from that. My mom not accepting what I had began to blame Jessica. My mom and Jessica had never gotten along. She began to believe that Jessica had put me under some sort of spell. Many of my relatives believe in witchcraft, and that only made my mom believe more in her nonsense. Anyways, being my parents, I accepted their way of finding a cure. With tears in our eyes we left the doctor's office that day. The very next morning my parents took me to see a curandero. A curandero is someone who treats witchcraft. They say that they cure through prayer and herbs. Some people call it black magic. I don't believe in this nonsense, but since it was my parent's way to cure me I saw the curandero. He lived in small crowded room. Every time I saw him he would give me some sort of drink that contained egg and some sort of herbs. It was slimy going down but it didn't have a bad taste. Then he would ask me to lie on the ground and he would message my back and my belly with a home made oil. He would be praying while he did this. I must have seen him about 5 times before I told my parents that he was only stealing their hard earned money. I had not been feeling any better and asked my parents to take me to see Dr. Skinner.

Even though it was very hard to see my self in a situation like that, I accepted what I had. Unfortunately, for my mom it was only a nightmare that she wanted to wake up from. By the time I got to see Dr. Skinner my condition had not improved. As a matter of fact, my skin felt like it was on fire and most of the numbness had become stiffness. My upper body was so numb that it felt like I was tightly wrapped with bandages. My chest area felt so tight that it made it very hard to breathe. Taking a deep breath felt like I was going to explode. Fortunately, I did not pop. Not only was my upper body affected, but my lower body as well. My calves, my thighs, and every other legs muscle felt so tight that walking became extremely difficult. Being carried around in a wheel chair is not funny especially when your legs feel like their going to pop from any movement that you try making. What made it more difficult was that mentally I felt fine. I had never asked for help, and even though it was hard to believe, this was no exemption. Dr. Skinner prescribed me amitriptyline. Amitriptyline is a drug used to treat depression. I was taking it because of the side effects. According to the doctor, it would relax me and make the numbness disappear. When I thought that things could not get any worse....they did. Soon after seeing Dr. Skinner my eyes became hypersensitive to the light. I was scared because I was quickly loosing my sight. Everybody who I looked at appeared to have this bright light shinning from behind them. It was as if they had a halo standing behind them. It was very difficult to make out who was in front of me. I immediately contacted Dr. Skinner and she recommended that I see an ophthalmologist. I was quickly loosing my sight, and fearing for my life I asked her if she knew an ophthalmologist. Luckily, she did, and that same day I got to see him. His name I don't remember out the back of my head, but I liked him. He examined my eyes thoroughly but could not find anything wrong. He ordered MRIs to be taken. The next day we went to his office, were he told me that he would be sending the MRIs to Dr. Skinner, and that I should see her for the explanation of why I almost could not see. That same day I called Dr. Skinner, and asked her if she would be able to see me. The following day we went to see her. Luckily, she had received the MRIs and began to explain why I could barely see. She told me that the nerves sending the images to my brain were not working properly, and allowed too much light to enter the brain. I asked her if I would ever be able see again. She responded by saying that my sight would improve as my condition improved. She also said that I would probably never see 20/20 again. My eyes were so sensitive to light that I proffered to keep my eyes closed. That same day I asked her for a drug that would improve my condition.

She began by explaining that she would first prescribe me a steroid, and once I had the M.S. under control we would begin the treatment. So, she prescribed me Prednisone. This steroid, even though a dangerous one, would make me stronger. I would take seven pills for 6 days and then one pill less every second day. Not only was I beginning to feel stronger, but I also gained about 50 pounds in the process.

What Happened with Magda?

When I began to loose my sight, not only was I numb, and weak but also depression began to settle in my head. I felt lost and the thoughts in my head were unhealthy. I felt like there was no point in living. I felt alone and in the dark. I became so depress that I wanted to sleep and never wake up. I began to wish I was dead. Not only was I screaming to my parents, my brothers, but also at every one else who would worry about me. Unfortunately, that included Magda. She would call me every night to see how I was doing, but also to wish me a good night. One night I just could not take it, and I threw my anger at her. I screamed at her, and asked her not to waste her time on me. I had screamed at her and began to wish that I had not done that. I hanged up and began to cry. I wanted her bad and now it seemed too late for me. Just minutes after hanging up on her she called back. "I hate you", she said and then hung up. I cried some more and began to regret becoming the trash I now had become. Even though I had screamed at her she called me every night to wish me a good night. One of those nights I asked her to take me out for fresh air. After weeks of being home resting on my bed. I needed to get out. She said that she would take me out only if my parents approved. So, I did what every independent man in my situation would do…I begged and then begged some more. It took a while, but I was able to convince them. The following day Magda's beautiful hands knocked at my door. With her help, I got to her car. She asked me where I wanted to go. I told her that I only wanted to get out of my house. She took me to the "Block" a nearby open mall. With her help I dragged my dead body around and rested quite often. Believe it or not, I felt great in her arms, so great that we took pictures of the afternoon. I did my best not to think of my problems. It was hard but she made it easy to enjoy the afternoon. We sat down and enjoyed a cup of hot chocolate that she had purchased at "Starbucks". Feeling better than past days I asked, "would you like to be my girlfriend?" she did not take long to answer. "Yes" she said, "But from now on you have to promise that we are going to get through this." I promised that I was going to give it my best. At that very moment I tasted the soft taste of nectar in her lips. It was a great night for me, a cold one, but a great one. From that moment on her strength and support made my suffering days worth it.

Our relationship began to grow and love began to emerge. My attitude towards life changed and once again I had something to live for. Even though I was facing some of the worst times in my life, she made every second worth it.

My Treatment

By Dr. Skinner's orders I was taking Amytriptaline for the numbness in my body, and Prednisone for my weakness. After gaining almost 50 pounds, little by little I began to walk by my self. My sight began to improve, but I had to wear dark sunglasses to protect my eyes from the light. I began to loose my balance. To make matters worse, my reflects were not responding properly. I was not capable to stand for a long time because it felt like I was on the roller coaster from hell. It only made things worse. Unfortunately, the side effects of the steroid were not pretty. I was covered by water bubbles that looked like pimples. Furthermore, my belly and arms were covered with stretch marks. I was getting stronger. After months of not being able to lift a glass of water I began getting the idea that everything was going to get back to normal. I was wrong. Once I stopped taking the steroids

I began to loose the strength that I had gained. I also began to loose my confidence. I must have been speaking with Dr. Skinner almost every day because once I told her what was going on; she immediately asked me to go in for Solimedrole infusions. Solimedrole is an ivy steroid that would take my body an hour to consume. The infusion center was located in the basement of the hospital. For five days I went to the infusion center where I saw people being treated for all sorts of cancers. Some of them had lost their hair; others were so weak that they needed personal assistance. The sight was not pretty. I began to say to my self that I did not belong in the same room. The Solimedrole was working. My strength began to grow stronger and stronger. I began to attend physical therapy. Soon my walking improved. My sight was improving, the stiffness turned into numbness, and the hypersensitivity in my skin decreased. Unfortunately, the effects of the Solimedrole only lasted a few weeks. I told Dr. Skinner what was happening, and she immediately placed me back on Solimedrole for what I hoped was going to be the last time. So, I am now a bit stronger, the stiffness is turning into numbness, and my sight is slowly improving. My reflects were the one symptom that was not improving. When the doctor hits my kneecap with that hammer like instrument I react by kicking a couple times. It is not a kick like you are use to. It is weird; my knees seem to jerk. It twitches in an indescribable way. My right knee reacts by jerking more than my left knee. My balance continues without any improvement. If I close my eyes I am not able to find my nose with my index finger. I also struggle on my feet.

I began to see a therapist for my physical functions. With help I practiced movements for my right hand, and practiced my walking. The second infusion of Solimedrole was working. My right hand began to function again but it now felt like a claw. I was able to grasp things but it only appeared like I was moving my thumb, middle finger, and pinky. My hand looked deformed; I had a three fingered claw. I was just happy I was able to use my right hand again. Physical therapy began to become easier. Soon my walking improved, and my balance problems began to improve. I was now attending physical therapy three times per week. The hypersensitivity in my body improved and I began to wear a larger variety of clothes. After being stuck with shorts and sweats, this was a big relief. Shortly after that, my reflects began to show signs of improvement. Unfortunately, I began to have tremor problems. I did not let the shaking get to me. Everything was going the way I wanted it to go. Even though it took a lot of begging I began to drive again. I remember that the first thing I did was to surprise Magda at her job with a couple of roses.

Soon, after seeing that exercise was the way to improvement I began to attend the gym. Even though, I was still suffering from my symptoms I made it a priority to improve. At first it was very difficult, but pound by pound my strength grew larger. I went from not being able to lift a glass of water to lifting a 20-pound weight in just 5 months of hard work. Physical therapy became too easy and I stopped attending. The gym became my only therapy, and to think that physical activities are a weakness. I also began to improve my dieting. I began to eat more fruit, nuts, and vegetables. "You are what you eat." This common saying began to make sense. My eating habits changed dramatically, although Dr. Skinner had not placed me on any special diet.

If I wanted to get better, it was only up to me to see that happen.

My confidence got stronger, my mind matured, and my body was once again strong. Even though, I had only regain enough strength to do simple activities I was going to give M.S., a fight to remember. I was going to the gym every day, and I only began to feel better. I had regained a small amount of movement in my right hand, and the hypersensitivity decreased to a point that I was able to stand. Many of the people, who daily fight M.S., learn to use their weak side of their body for daily activities. The reason why this happens is simply because M.S. affects more the stronger side of the body. That means that if you are a right-hander you need to learn to become a southpaw, and by versa. I did exercises for my right hand everyday. I would squeeze a stress ball. After almost 2 years of doing that I regained strength in my hand and everything became easier. In the mean time I learned how to deal with my struggles by learning to use my left hand. Soon brushing my teeth became easier, and eating sure became easier as well. Tying my shoes was still difficult, but I was getting some where with all of my hard work. I don't understand why but I was not loosing any weight. I was going to the gym and sweating like a dog on a summer day. For the first time in a long time I began to feel victorious. I was little by little becoming more independent and it felt great. My coordination and balance were at a point were I was able to control it. The shaking was not improving, but I was just glad that I was taking control of my body again. Although nothing felt right I knew that I was going to survive. I wanted to be normal so I kept fighting.

My Inspiration

My relationship with Magda was only getting better. Since I was now able to drive I was able to see her every day. We were in love. We were having a good time, especially because she made me have fun, something that I had not experience in a long time. My attitude towards life changed. It was no longer about surviving but about living with a smile on my face. I learned that it was not a bout winning the battle but winning the war. The shyness that I suffered from during my younger years disappeared. I became more outgoing and spoke my mind. A new Edwin had been born.

My new loving attitude surprised everyone. I was no longer the outsider. It felt great to feel involved again. I had gotten most of my symptoms under control. I was stronger, but still suffered from the hypersensitivity in my body and my eyes, and the numbness was slowly banishing. Through my hard work and the support I received from every body I was defeating this strange but interesting phenomenon. I continued to get my ass to gym every day hoping that one day I will be normal again.

Dr. Skinner decided that it was time to begin treatment. Even though it is not a cure it is a start. I was placed on Avonex. Avonex is a drug, an expensive one, which is to be self-administered once a week. That meant that I had to have an injection once a week. The first couple of times I tried to inject it my self. I should have never done that because it hurts like you can't imagine. From that moment on, my dad began to inject me, and to this day pain is not a factor. Avonex for most people is a re-energizer because it makes every day easier. I have not experience that effect yet, and I think that it is because I am young and I have a fighting attitude. The package contains a month supply that will shrink your bank account $1100 every month.

Even though, my conditions has gradually improved I could not wait to start looking for a job. After almost a year of being out of commission Dr. Skinner allowed me to seek employment. I had to wear dark sunglasses everywhere that I went, but I was just happy to be out in the open. Anyways I loved my new look. The hypersensitivity was under control and soon I became used to it. Some of the numbness in my body had almost banished. My feet remained numb, but soon I became used to it. My balance problem had diminish along with my reflect problems. Although I had 17/20 vision I felt great. I was very enthusiastic about getting back in the work force. I was tired of resting and receiving disability insurance that barely paid my bills. I had to pay $400 a month for my car, plus car insurance, my health insurance my medicine, and frankly $220 a week was not enough.

You may be asking why my parents did not help me out with my bills. The reason is because ever since I've had a job I don't allow anybody to help me financially, no matter how deep of a problem I'm in. Although they are my parents, I did not feel comfortable asking them for money.

My first stop of course was the Orange County Teachers Federal Credit Union. Surprised about my accomplishment they did not hesitate to re-hire me on the spot. I said hello to everybody that knew me at work.

Followed by the saying, "guess who is back?" I was glad to be back to work, and to have made a difference. During the time that I was gone, OCTFCU changed their benefit requirements. Now you only needed to work for one month before earning the right to your benefits. If you remember, it used to be three months.

Once again I was back on the road. For how long, who knows? To avoid stress I began to take tai-chi. I also decided that I was going to take some more time off from school and focus on my well being. I began by working part-time. They were not that many new faces in my team, but every day I said good morning and good night to every individual. Many asked me what had happen and I took the time to explain it to every body. I began to live life with a smile.

"What doesn't kill you only makes you stronger." This saying became my motto. Still going to the gym, I gave 110% of effort every day. I tried to live life to the fullest even if it meant staying after work. I was proud to work with my team. I made great friends there. We had a great time playing pranks on each other. It was a great time in my life. Not knowing how I was going to wake up every morning, I continued to force my self into going to work and having fun. I forgot to mention that M.S. wears you down every single day. I needed to rest, not sleep, 10 hours every night. At first that seemed impossible but after a while it became a piece of cake. Believe it or not there is a difference between rest and sleep. I discovered that rest was more valuable than sleep. When I rested I felt re-energized and ready to go while sleeping only lead to tiredness. Every morning was a fight because like every one I too had my bad days, days where fatigue seemed hard to hide. There were days where my sight was affected more, and even days where getting up seemed impossible. No matter how bad of a day I was having; I never showed up to work with a grinch on my face. Every day became about having fun and forgetting my problems. I got to see Magda every night after work. She made my efforts worth it.

Her pretty smile always waited for me to arrive and take her out for coffee or hot chocolate. Every night I would see her and with every single one of her tender kisses I would touch the stars. Every day that I saw her was like falling in love over and over again. What I loved about our relationship was that my mom liked her. Our love grew, and continued to grow every day. On February 14, 2003, Valentines Day, I took Magda to the beach. It was there that while walking under the light of the moon I got down on one knee and asked her to marry me. She helped me up and responded with a sincere yes. We kissed and forgot about the freezing water that reached our ankles. That night became the happiest night of my life, and my inspiration to keep fighting.

The One

Even though, nothing felt normal, I was sure that Magda was the one. She was the backbone of our relationship, and my recovery. She had helped me through the rough ride I had just experienced. I was very proud of my self because what I had accomplished was no easy task. I was also in love, and engaged to the woman of my dreams. I was beating M.S. and had returned to work. I was briefly back on my feet and living life one day at a time. Maintaining multiple sclerosis under control was very difficult. When you are dealing with M.S. there is no way of knowing how you will be feeling the next day. You have to put up a fight every morning because the fight you won yesterday wants a rematch. Every morning in my life is different because I never know what I will be dealing with tomorrow. The struggle could be caused by anything. My skin may be more hypersensitive than ever. I may feel weaker, I may also be blind. My balance could be worse, my reflects could not be responding properly, and I can even wake up number than what I have become used to. The numbness in my body never disappeared completely, but I have adapted to feeling my limbs numb. My right hand remains to feel stiff, but with hard work I now have movement. My left hand is now my dormant hand, even though little by little I have regained some strength in my right hand. Dr. Skinner was surprised with my recovery because she had never seen a recovery as quick as mine. I may have been out of commission for about a year, but from what she told me: the usual recovery takes other people about 18 months. Although my recovery was quick what surprised her the most was that I regained strength and movement in my right hand. She says that many of her patients never recover strength or movement in their limbs as well as I have. Although, I had recovered, simple tasks remain to be a challenge. For example, the stiffness in my right hand prevents me from feeling confident at work. The stiffness doesn't allow me to have much feeling, and when working with currency I have to be more careful. I can no longer type and using the computer with one hand feels uncomfortable. The movement in my right hand is not great. Tying my shoes remains a challenge. I can no longer depend on my right hand for support. I cannot trust my hand because I don't know how much strength I am using or need to use. My feet are also numb, and it is because of that reason that loosing my balance is a simple task. Although I can walk, not being careful on what I step on can cause me to kiss the floor. I can no longer run or jog. Walking fast is a bit hard but I manage as long as I do not slip or trip over my feet. Stepping up or down the stairs is very difficult if there is no hand rail. My walking is not always right. There are days when my legs feel so weak that walking becomes difficult. Sometimes it is one leg, sometimes it is both, but my fighting attitude puts me on my feet. I go to work even if I have to drag my dead leg behind me. I may not be walking properly but being at work makes me forget of my problems. No matter what my condition is I always have a smile on my face. I live one day at a time, and always seeking for fun. Management at OCTFCU has told me several times that I put the un in fun and that work is not the same when I am not there. I make work fun whether I am feeling well or not. I make jokes or just play pranks on my team members. One of my favorite pranks was telling my supervisor to be careful because she could trip over her shoe lasses. She would bend down to tie her shoe lasses. When she realized that she was wearing high heels. The reason why I wake up every morning is because I am going to have fun no matter where I am. I have learned that life is lived one day at a time, and that there is no tomorrow.

Although, I am not attending school for the moment I do plan to return to school one day. For now I am only focusing on my well being, and my new life. I keep a strict no fast food diet, and I exercise regularly. I continue to attend the gym a minimum of three times per week. I take M.S. to the next level by discovering new things that I can no longer do, and by creating a new way of doing those things. I always say, "If I am not able to do it today. I may be able to do it tomorrow, and if not tomorrow, the day after". Living with multiple sclerosis has taught me to never give up no matter how hard it may seem.

No matter how bad my condition may seem I am not disabled. It may appear hard to believe, but my fighting attitude doesn't allow me to miss a day from work. As long as I can stand on my feet, I will always get my ass to work. I love my work. I love assisting members, suggesting products that will better their financial status, and of course, to put a smile on their faces. I do my best to try to make the Member's day a good one. I love the people who I work with, and it is the fun that we have together that inspires me every morning not to give up on my fight to beat the interesting phenomena that I live with. Not knowing what weakness I am going to be dealing with tomorrow is a disadvantage. A disadvantage because, I have no idea what will help me survive. I have adapted to the hypersensitivity in my body, but there are those days when it is intolerable and it makes everything that touches me painful. There are days when maintaining my balance is like trying to keep a roller coaster from speeding and turning. There are days when death seems like the only solution. Although, the gym has slowly help me regain some of my strength I am still weaker than before. I now have lived with M.S. for about two years, and I still cannot bench press more than half my weight. I used to weigh 190 pounds, and after two long years of exercise I now weigh 240 pounds. Although, I am not satisfied with my weight I could be in a worse situation. Getting up every morning is difficult but at least I am able to get up.

I may be sick, but I am not dieing. I may struggle on my feet, but it is only up to me to not give up. Multiple sclerosis may impair me from many things but living is not one of them. Multiple sclerosis is not going to kill me; unfortunately it will make it easier for any virus or bacteria to enter my body. It will also make it harder for me to recover from any other sicknesses. Fortunately, I have only had to deal with the flu a couple of times. It may have taken me 3 weeks to recover, but I am just happy that it did not kill me. For me the flu always was a two-day dilemma. Unfortunately, dealing with the flu for three weeks was not pretty. Nothing worked, and chicken soup did not help one bit. The coughing was so bad that I sounded like an elephant calling for help. My nose was so runny that no roller coaster would be able to catch up to it. Fighting the flu kept me from attending work, but during that time I feared of having a relapse. Luckily for me I was able to return to work once the flu lost its strength.

Although it was very hard to attend work my attitude towards life earned me a lot of respect. Respect may not be much for many people, but for me it was like being on top of the world. My dedication to my health allowed me to touch the hearts of others. Even though, I was able to keep most of my symptoms under control the tremor problems were making me feel uncomfortable at work. I was shaking enough to make the members that I was assisting ask me if I was okay. That question soon became common, too common, and I asked Dr. Skinner to prescribe me a drug to help with my tremor problems. You may be asking why I didn't ask for it sooner, and the reason why is because I do not like to be on medication. I hate taking pills, and the only reason why I inject Avonex into my system was because they say that it helps me, although, they say that patients on Avonex have less severe exacerbations, relapses. I feel no change after administering it. I think that the reason why I feel no change after taking Avonex is because I am young and willing to fight. Avonex acts like a re-energizer for other patients, but remember other patients are usually older and weaker. No doctor really understands why I have to deal with M.S. Remember; multiple sclerosis is more common in older people. Almost 90% of all patients are older than 30, and almost 65% of those cases are woman. It is safe to say that I am dealing with a rare case of M.S., but rare or not I was chosen for a reason. It may be a disadvantage, however I will overcome it. It can be a lesson that will open my eyes to something that many people cannot see. Maybe, just maybe, one day the tables will turn, and I will have the advantage. Hope is what keeps me alive. I have the faith that one day there will be a cure, and that day I hope to have the advantage on everyone else.

My symptoms may be under some sort of control. I continue to attend work daily and the gym at least three nights after work. I have earned the respect I deserve. The Teachers Credit Union has awarded me with beautiful trophies for my teamwork, leadership, and the great service I provided. For the very first time in two years I felt extremely happy and filled with joy. I was beginning to have success in life, again. My professional life at OCTFCU was great, but my personal life was also at its best.

Magda and I had set the wedding to take place on a clear November afternoon. We were going to get married at Picnic Beach in Laguna Niguel. I had told my parents who were shocked at first, but approved of our intentions. I don't clearly understand why Magda refused to let me ask her mom for her hand in marriage. Magda's dad died when she was a little girl, so asking her mom was the right thing to do. She never actually told her mom of our plans. She said that she was waiting for the right time, unfortunately after a month of engagement I began to pressure her because I did not feel right for her mom to find out a day before the wedding. One afternoon we got into a big argument, and we stopped talking to each other for a couple of days. We came to an agreement, and things returned to normal. October came around, and her mom still did not know. I became very upset with her because that was not part of our agreement. With the wedding being a month away I had a relapse. The wedding was cancelled, and a new date has not been set.

The Second Time Around

Very upset with what had happen I began to focus on my recovery. Doctor Skinner took me off of work. Luckily for me the law protected me and I did not have to resign. Once again weakness took over my body, and walking became difficult. The hypersensitivity once again became uncomfortable. The old sweats and short once again became my wardrobe. Luckily, I did not loose my eyesight. I became more hypersensitive to the light, but my sight was not harmed as long as I wore dark lenses. Numbness was all over my body. Soon it became stiffness. Stiffness that was worse than before. I was so stiff that I felt no hunger. My stomach was numb enough for me to feel no hunger. When I needed to use the throne there was no way for me to know if I was done. Not attending work meant that I had more time to exercise. Since my legs felt stiff maintaining my balance was very difficult. Dr. Skinner recommended that I start using a cane for assistance, but I didn't even think of doing so. My strength was once again overwhelmed by this strange disorder. My hard work had meant nothing. Once again I was back to the beginning. Once again Dr. Skinner placed me on Prednisone. The steroid was doing its job, and I began to regain some of my lost strength. I went almost a whole year without having a relapse. It was a battle that had started all over again. Most patients with M.S. have relapses every six months. I was able to keep M.S. under control for almost a year, and for me that was a great accomplishment. Like the first time I was taking Amitriptalyne for the numbness, and I continued to inject my self with Avonex. I was taking a high dosage of Prednisone, and after a month I was back on my feet. Just after two weeks of being off the steroid I began to loose some of my strength. I contacted Dr. Skinner, and she placed me on Solimedrole. Once again I had to go to the infusion center that I never wanted to visit again. I was there for an hour everyday for a whole week. The Solimedrole did its job, and my exercise routine became something that I was able to accomplish. My routine consists of walking a mile no matter how I may be walking. During my relapse it took me 45 minutes to walk a mile rather than the 25 minutes that it was taking me during my previous fight with M.S. My routing also consists of butterflies, arm extensions, leg extensions, arm/leg curls, leg press, and abdominal exercises.

During my relapse my left hand began to feel like my right hand. Loosing strength and loosing movement in my left hand I began to worry. I was terrified of the idea that I had no good hand to really depend on. My tremor problems were worst, so bad that I could not lift a glass of water without making a spill. I had no dominant hand, and every day activities became very difficult. A new symptom emerged I began to feel a tingly sensation in my face. I was very worried because I did not want to have more problems. Fortunately, that tingly sensation didn't last long. As my condition began to improve some of the stiffness disappeared, and my left hand became more flexible and moveable. Not having complete control in my hands I returned to work in late January of 2004. It took me almost four months, but I was back on my feet. I had pushed my self beyond my limits to return to work. I felt very happy to be back to work; however it did not feel right. My tremor problems had improved, but not having complete feeling in my hands made my job difficult. My hands felt like I had cut the circulation of blood, and felt numb and huge. Just like when you fall a sleep on your hands. My feet remained so numb that movement felt tingly. The numbness and lack of complete movement in my hands made me feel uncomfortable dealing with currency and using a computer. I spoke with Tracy, my supervisor and a good friend, about the difficulty I was having. She said that I should try to relax and that maybe I should talk with my doctor. Tracy was very supportive, every morning she would ask me how I was feeling. Anyways, I got to see Dr. Skinner and she recommended that a brief vacation would probably be the best solution. She said that I was recovering from a relapse, and that it was probably the best time for me to enjoy a relaxing vacation. She was right. Mentally I felt great, and I began to believe that if I didn't take advantage of traveling I would probably never have the opportunity again. I felt strong, and the doctor agreed. I had to find a way to relax and enjoy life to the fullest. The following day I spoke with Tracy, and the rest of the management team. I told them that I was working so hard to beat M.S. that it became my only priority. I told them that I was tired of work after work, after work, and that I needed to dedicate some time to my self. I let them know that, that week would be my last one. I told them that I needed to do something that I had never done before. I had decided that I was going to travel and explore new grounds.

New Grounds

That night when I got home I told my parents
of my plans to travel. I was expecting them to
be alarmed and terrified of the idea. However,
they took me by surprise when they agreed
with me. They said that the past two years had
been very hard for me, and I probably needed
some time to relax and enjoy. By the following
day every team member at work knew that I
was leaving. They asked why? I simply told
them that I needed to do something that I
would probably never have the opportunity of
doing by my self again. They all wished me the
best wishes and that my story had touched the
darkest place in their hearts. That weekend I
was on a plane to Acapulco.

Magda's grandfather had been very sick,
and his last wishes were to see everybody
together again. Magda had not seen her grandfather for almost 10 years. So she and her
mother got on a plane to Zitacuaro,

Michoacan in Mexico. Our flights were only a couple of days apart. Anyways, I was arriving to Acapulco with no one of my family members in Chilpancingo knowing. Remember that Chilpancingo is only miles from Acapulco. I only told one of my cousins that I was going to be arriving soon. He told me that Miriam, my cousin, was having her Quinseanera in two days. I decided to surprise her on that special day. I had not spoken to her in almost three years and I being there was going to freak her out. Denny, my cousin, picked me up at the airport. I asked him not to tell anyone that I was there. I wanted it to be a surprise for everyone. He told me that Miriam would be very happy of me attending her Quinseanera. A Quinseanera is the celebration of her 15th birthday similar to the sweet sixteen here in the U.S. Nobody knew that I was going to be there. For a whole day I avoided making contact with anybody that knew me. When the party was ready to begin I waited for my beautiful cousin and family in the entrance to the church. You see, the celebration first begins by attending a special mass. It was great, seeing her in her beautiful light, pastel purple dress run towards me. It made me feel great. With a spring in her step she got to me, and greeted me with a humongous kiss. It felt wonderful. She was speechless and all because of me. All of my family members were going to be there, and when they saw me they thought that they were seeing a ghost. It was great. They knew the situation I was in and never thought that I would be traveling by my self. After greeting everyone it was time for the party. We carpooled to the salon, where we were greeted by mariachis. We then took our seats and the celebration began. The food was great. There was live music as well as a dj. The party lasted almost all night. I had not dance in a long time, and to be honest with you I thought that with the balance problems I was having I would not be able to move my feet at a fast pace. I loved to dance. Before my diagnoses I was a good salsa and merengue dancer. Miriam asked me to dance with her, and I could not say no to her. So step by step I slowly got into rhythm. Even though, I got tired very quickly I enjoyed the moment. When it got time to get some rest, every one wanted to take me home with them. I had many choices, and it was very hard to make up my mind. Although it took me some time I finally decided that I would go back to Denny's place; where I had my baggage. It was about 4 o'clock in the morning when I finally got to bed. For the first time in a very long time, I had no desire to be in bed. When morning came I went to have breakfast with my grandmother. Unfortunately, she did not recognize me. She is 95 years old, and she is beginning to forget. To me it did not matter. We had breakfast, and then she remembered who I was. It made me feel really good to have put a smile on her wrinkled, but beautiful face. That morning I felt extremely tired, and fatigued. I spent the remaining hours of the morning sleeping. When I woke up it was about 2 o'clock. The remaining hours of the day I spent answering questions rewarding my condition. After that day no one else asked. It was great since I had left the U.S. to try to forget and relax. I spent one whole month in Chilpancingo. During that time I visited some beautiful places. I went to the humongous cathedral located in the centro or downtown. My cousins took me to the manantiales, the waterfall, located only 45 minutes from Chilpancingo. I was afraid of getting in the water. I had not swum in 2 years, and frankly I was scared. I had no idea of how my condition would react to the water. After my cousins insisted I finally got into the water. It felt great. While I was in the water I felt normal. When it got time to leave, I did not want to get out of the water. During my stay in Chilpancingo I was able to maintain the M.S. under control. My main problem was the bright days. Even though, I was wearing my dark shades there were times when they didn't help much. Furthermore, my stay there was great. I stopped taking the tremor drugs that Dr. Skinner had prescribed me. I began to shake less. I felt more relax, and I was for once enjoying my life. I knew the phone number of where Magda was staying. We were in contact every other day. We arranged a vacation. The plans made me feel very happy, and enthusiastic. I was looking forward to our upcoming adventure. My first stop was in Zitacuaro, where Magda was staying. My cousin took the long 6 hour bus ride with me. When we got to Zitacuaro we stayed at the Hotel Mexico. It was a very nice hotel. Clean, a big room, and very nice people that provided many services. The first thing I did was to call Magda, and let her know that I was in town. That afternoon she came to the hotel. There she met my cousin. Then we went out for a walk. My cousin left the next day because he needed to get back to school. I was on my own and independent again. I saw Magda every single day. We began to make arrangements for our vacation together. Our plans were to travel around Mexico. Our first stop was going to be Huatulco then Yucatan and finally Cancun. Then she was going to meet my family members in Chilpancingo before returning to Zitacuaro. Zitacuaro was very calm and beautiful. It reminded me of Chilpancingo. I was feeling great. The weather was different and it gave me an advantage on the M.S. I had most of the symptoms under control. It was hard to get up in the morning, but once I was on my feet everything became easier. Every morning I felt very tired and fatigued. I did not understand why? I was getting about 9 hour of sleep every night. During my time in Zitacuaro, the weather was pleasant. The days were about 75 degrees and the sun was not so bright. I learned that Magda's grandfather had been hospitalized, and was very ill. Magda no longer felt enthusiastic about our plans, I noticed it in her face one day. She was not her happy self, and I told her it was okay if she wanted to stay with her family. A few days later I learned that he past away. On the eight day I kissed Magda goodbye and left. It was very hard because I was looking forward to traveling with Magda by my side. I felt heart-broken, even though I was the one who told her that she should stay.

The Road to Happiness

My first stop was Huatulco, Oaxaca. To get there I took two buses. Even though, the ride took about 4 long hours I enjoyed the hot climate in Huatulco. I only stayed one day in Huatulco because spring break was soon to arrive and all the flights to Yucatan were booked. Huatulco is a beautiful bay. The warm climate made it very difficult to stay away from the shoreline. Huatulco is a beautiful city. You were able to take advantage of many great activities that the small quiet city offers. The sand was a beautiful golden brown color. The water was a bit cold, but felt great. The only thing that I did here was relax by the water. The next day I was on a plane to Yucatan. Since I was flying out from Mexico City I took a short bus ride to Mexico City. When I arrived at the airport it was probably

10 o'clock in the morning. Since my flight was going to depart at 3 o'clock I began to wonder around the airport. I was hungry so I began to look for a place where I could eat. I entered the first place that I found. It was a small deli. I ordered the worst tasting ham and cheese sandwich that I have ever tasted. I complained, of course, but after not gaining anything from it. I had no choice but to stop the noises my stomach was making. Later I learned that a Burger King was located at the other side of the airport. It was only 12 o'clock, and I had to find a way to kill time, so I began to wonder around the huge, spacious, and luxurious airport. By 2:45 I had explored the entire airport, and had entered almost every shop in the busy airport. My flight was 40 minutes late, and the anxiety to get to Merida, Yucatan's capital, just seemed to grow bigger and bigger.

It was only a two hour flight. When I finally arrived in Yucatan I took a taxi tour of Merida. The tour took a few hours, but it was worth the $100 pesos that I spent for the tour. Merida is a beautiful city, especially at night. It has beautiful gardens and a square plaza unlike the round plazaz that most cities have. After the tour, it was probably 8 o'clock and I had no hotel to settle in. I asked the taxi driver to take me to a hotel located by the coast. He took me to Progresso. He said that Progresso was a quiet, calm city located on the coast with the Gulf of Mexico. It was a drooling 45 minute drive from Merida to Progresso, and it was also the most expensive taxi ride that I had ever paid for. $460 pesos. However, when I got to Progresso the $45 dollars that I paid were worth it. Progresso is a beautiful small town that is filled with many activities to pass the time. I stayed at the Tropical Suites hotel located across the street from the beach. The environment in Progresso is great. Everyone seemed very friendly, curious, and caring. You only needed to walk in the sand to understand why the people were so happy. Walking in the warm sand was a challenge for me. It was difficult because unlike the sidewalk when you step onto the sand you begin to sink. Although, it was difficult to maintain my balance in the sand I managed to make my way to the warm, clear blue water. By the second day my legs became very sore. I had only been in Progresso for a couple of days, but I was convinced that life by the sea was great. The ocean water is so clean that it sparkled. It was so clear that you were able to see your reflection in the water. The water was a bit warmer than any other beach, but with the warm climate it felt great. The sun rose at about 6 o'clock every morning, and slowly hid around 7 o'clock in the evening. The sky was clean, as well as the fresh air and with no clouds in sight the days were wonderful. The days were warm, very warm, but pleasant as long as you did not forget to apply sunscreen. If you like seafood you will love the variety of dishes that Progresso offers. The fish, as well as other sea creatures, is fresh since it is fished daily, and cooked in many delicious ways. The service in the restaurants is clean, and friendly. Your food is prepared your way and served in the soft, brown, and clean sand of the beach. If you are a Margarita lover, like me, you will love enjoying the cold drink under the shade of a palm tree.

The air is fresh, and runs almost all day. Unfortunately, the nights were warm, and I found it difficult to rest with the air conditioner turned on. In Progresso life is simple. The town is very busy by sunrise, but appears like a ghost town once the sun begins to kiss the day goodbye. Vendors are everywhere from the shore to the streets. People are just trying to make a living, and many times if you are patient you will get a good deal. Whether you are renting jet skis or purchasing an artifact the perfect price comes up if you make an offer. If you find communicating in Spanish difficult don't worry because most vendors know some English. Believe it or not, most people in Progresso are retired Americans or people who are just taking a break from the real world, like me. If you decide to walk to El Centro, down-town, you will notice that it is very busy, and a bit crowded. What I loved about Progresso is that it was only a 15 minute walk from the beach to El Centro. The town is very safe. Everywhere that you turn you will see police officers. When you get to downtown you will notice that many of the buildings are similar in structure to those in the U.S. The mall or centro comercial as they call it here, are just like the ones back in the states. Many of the stores are what I like to call Americanized. What I mean is that you can purchase many American products for a decent price. So don't panic if you forget to pack your shaving gel, toothpaste, or any other item because you can purchase it here.

Progresso is a great place. It has a great atmosphere, and it is a great place to relax, forget, and have fun. They're many fun things to do in this small, quiet town. Like I mentioned earlier life by the sea is great. Nice weather, a clean beach, and many activities to pass the time. You can take a tour around the town and beaches. Furthermore, you can rent a small boat, jet skis, skates, bikes, and even mopeds. If you like you can snorkel, dive, swim, and even parasail. Progresso is a beautiful town to visit. It is not an expensive vacation. Everything is pretty much economical. My hotel room was only $250 pesos a night, about $23 dollars per night.

On my last day something very strange happened. It was Wednesday; it was also my 21st birthday, the day started like every other day. However, on this Wednesday the beach, and even downtown appeared to be deserted. The restaurants were open. The stores were open, but no one was buying. It felt lonely, as if I had the entire town to myself. The weather was also different. The wind was blowing a bit stronger than usual. It was still a bit warm, but on this day they were puffy gray clouds covering the blue sky.

After 5 days in Progresso my stay came to an end. My stay in Progresso was great. I enjoyed relaxing, and drinking a Margarita every afternoon under the shade of a palm tree. It was time for me to move on, and write a new page in my life's journey. I am sure that I will visit the small, relaxing town in the future. Although, I enjoyed my stay in Yucatan there were days when the heat would provoke the hypersensitivity in my body. Some days I felt so weak that I only spent the day sitting under a palm tree. Luckily for me, I did not have problems with my sight. Although it was hard at first, I learned how to walk in the soft sand.

After a marvelous stay in Progresso I decided that I wanted to explore one of the best beaches that the Gulf of Mexico offers, Cancun. Since Cancun was only a 3 hour drive from Merida I decided that I was going to take the bus to Cancun. The next day I got up very early in the morning. I got on a bus to Merida. It only cost me $12 pesos to get from Progresso to Merida. After a boring 45 minute drive I bought a bus ticket to Cancun. Luckily, the next departure to Cancun was in 20 minutes. It was about 12:30 in the afternoon when I finally got to Cancun. I began to explore. So pulling my small baggage behind me I began to walk around the small centro. The first thing I noticed was that almost every single item had tripled in price. After wondering for a few hours I decided that it was time to find a hotel. So I got on a taxi, and asked the driver to take me to a hotel near the beach. After a 25 minute drive I finally got to see the beautiful water that sparkled like a diamond. The hotels were not what I was expecting. The gigantic resorts covered the entire shoreline. I asked the driver to stop in every resort so that I could find out the prices they were charging. One hotel charged $2000 pesos per night. Another charged $1800 pesos per night. I did not like the prices one bit, but I knew that I had no choice but to pay these horrifying prices. I did not give up, and 15 hotels later I was able to negotiate a fair price. I arrived at the Cancun Plaza resort there I was able to pay $1000 pesos per night for a room that would regularly cost $1500 big ones. In Cancun you can find any hotel that could be found in the States. Here in Cancun I was paying $1000 pesos for a room. While in Progresso I paid less than $300 pesos per night, and I was only a few steps from the beach. Although I was not happy with the price I was paying, the room had it all. A luxurious bathroom, walk-in closets, a small kitchen, king size bed, an amazing view of the beach, and a big screen television. For once I felt like a superstar living the luxurious life. After putting my belongings away I put on my bathing suite, and walked to the beach. Before reaching the ocean I stopped at the full service bar located by the pool. I ordered a margarita, which cost me $40 pesos, ten more pesos then in Progresso and was about half the size. I sipped down my margarita before getting to the beach. Anyways, when I got to the beach Progresso seemed like rocky mud. Cancun's water is crystal clear. It looks like you are entering an ocean filled with purified water. Unfortunately, the water was still salty, and the waves were a bit stronger. What I liked most about Cancun was that you were able to walk at least 85 yards into the water without having the water reach over your chin. I am only 5'11 and after walking 50 yards into the water, the clear water only reached my rib area. Although I found it very difficult to walk in the sand, the beach was wonderful. What made it difficult to walk was the sand because it feels like flour. The sand is beautiful. Not only white, but very soft as well. The sand is grained to perfection. Cancun's sand was like nothing I had ever seen before; it was like walking on flour. It feels like your sinking, so maintaining my balance was a big challenge. Although walking in the soft sand was difficult, I managed to get around. Walking in the soft sand felt very relaxing. While I was in Cancun I enjoyed listening to the wave's crash against the huge rocks found near the shore. Like in Progresso the weather in Cancun is great. The days are warm, sunny, and beautiful. Unlike Progresso the nights are cool. Like Progresso, Cancun also offers many fun activities. There is not many palm threes, and coconuts are not easy to find.

Let me give you a piece of advice. If you ever decide to travel to Cancun be prepare to spend. I say this because everything is expensive. Some items are even pricier than in the U.S. food is very expensive. While I was in Zitacuaro, I would pay $20 pesos for a hamburger and fries combo. In Progresso the same combo cost $25 pesos, but in Cancun it cost

$75 pesos. When you arrive in Cancun, I recommend that you rent a car because the resorts are separated from society. A car rental is the only thing that I did not find expensive. You can rent a car for about $250 pesos per day. Unfortunately, when I found out of this great deal it was too late. I recommend that you visit Isla Mujeres. Island of Woman is a gorgeous island located a few miles from shore. You might also make the effort to go to playa delfines, dolphin beach. One day I woke up at 5 o'clock in the morning, and then walked for almost two hours to get to playas mujeres. Let me tell you that the walk there was worth it because I got to see dolphins out in the open. Seeing them swim free made me feel very good, and seeing something like that is something I will never forget.

During my stay in Cancun it actually rained. That's right it rained, and for the first time in my life I found out how great it feels to swim while it rains. Although it was raining the climate felt warm. It was unbelievable. My stay in Cancun came to end. I wish that I would have had more time to spend in Cancun, but I had promised my family in Chilpancingo that I would return by April 9rd to celebrate my birthday. I had many bills to pay back home so a couple of more days in Cancun were not in my budget.

April 9th was a Saturday. That morning I woke up at 4 o'clock. My flight departed at 7:30 so I needed to get to the airport. The day before my departure I had asked the hotel manager to have a taxi ready for me at 5. Since I had no idea how far the airport was I needed to calculate my time carefully. Little did I know that the airport was only 20 minutes away. Since the streets were empty the taxi driver had no problem speeding to the airport. My flight departed right on time. By 9 o'clock I was in Mexico City. Then I took a boring hour taxi drive to the bus station. The next bus to Chilpancingo would be leaving at 11:30. Unfortunately, I was unable to get on that bus because all the tickets had been sold. I had to wait for the next bus, which would leave at 2 o'clock. I must have waited an eternity. Fortunately the bus left right on time. It was going to be a long three and a half hour bus ride that seemed very quick because I was watching The Matrix Reloaded on the bus theater system. When I finally got to Chilpancingo my cousins were at the bus station waiting for me. Since they knew that I would be traveling with Magda they were upset when I told them that my plans had changed because of an unexpected death in Magda's family. Anyways, the fiesta would be on the next day. The food preparations were ready and the guest list included every one who knew my name.

My aunt knew that I loved to wear suits, so she took me to see a tailor that sold suits. I was not expecting so many suits to choose from, but after a few minutes I found the perfect one. I had always wanted a white suit, so when I saw it I knew it had to be mine. I was surprised by the price. It only cost $400 pesos. I looked great in my new suit. Everybody loved it. When it came time to party I got to enjoy great food with the people I love. Everybody took pictures with me, and everybody looked very happy. The following week I passed most of the time talking about my adventures along the Mexican bay. I also showed everybody the pictures that I had brought back from my trip. Since my cousins were in town we planned a trip to Acapulco. So the following morning we were on our way to Acapulco, where we had a lot of fun hanging out. Acapulco is like hell, the sun burns the skin right off. The temperature is horrible. It is about 110 degrees during the day and about 80 degrees during the night making it impossible to sleep. I still enjoyed every minute of my stay there.

After returning to Chilpancingo I began packing my bags because it was time to return home and continue my fight to be happy. I had no job to return to, so I knew that I had some tough days ahead. However, I was relaxed and re-energized. I was ready for anything. After such a long time of relaxation my body felt great and I knew that I had to continue pushing. My long relaxing road trip taught me that there is more to life then suffering and that if we want something we have to go after it.

This trip showed me that the truth about life is happiness. It showed me that if we can find happiness within ourselves we can do anything no matter how difficult it may seem.

Primerica

As I returned back to the real world from such a long relaxing vacation I was energized and ready to go find out what I can make of myself. I applied for a position at OCTFCU, I had a great experience there so I really wanted to return there, but unfortunately they had no positions open so I kept on looking.

My cousin Dee had come in contact with Primerica, a financial services company. The recruiter wanted to hire her but she was confused about the job. She asked me to accompany her to a business briefing. I was overwhelmed with the type of work the company did that my cousin and I joined the company and became business partners.

Primerica is a big life insurance company that is part of Citi-group and also offers several services to increase cash flow. Products such as affordable life insurance, a SMART loan program (simple interest home loans that helps people payoff the mortgage and debt at a faster pace and also reduces taxes for the client).Furthermore, they also offer investments like retirement account and other investment accounts.

Soon after joining I got my life license and attended all of the seminars to assist me in understanding how the products help clients become debt free and increase their cash flow and even improve their life styles. I was really excited because I had the opportunity to make a difference in family's lives and the pay was great. Unfortunately the income was only commission base. I was not ready to commit full time to this line of work so I applied at the Orange County Credit Union (OCCU) where I was hired as a telephone service representative.

I was working part-time at OCCU and only worked on my Primerica duties when it came up. Since I was my own boss thru Primerica I did not have to worry about goals. As a matter of fact, during my time at OCCU I really did not work with Primerica.

After a year of working at OCCU late July of 2005 I decided that I deserved better, so I left and began working full time for Primerica.

Primerica offered me the opportunity to be my own boss and if everything went well my income could be tripled if not better.

I knew that it might take a few months before my business could take off so I was planning on living from the money that I had been saving.

Primerica gave me the opportunity to change my life style. I would not have to worry about being in the office at a certain time. I was in charge of when I wanted to work and when I wanted to rest. I was in charge and it was great.

I Know You!

Let me tell you a little bit more of how my life used to be, so that you can relate to my situation with more understanding. Like you know I was born in Los Angeles California, but grew up in a small town in Mexico. After moving back to the states my parents pressured me and my brother to become the best in school. In school I was the quiet one in the corner who never raised his hand and would only talk if I was spoken too.

I was very successful in school, and I owe it all to my perfect attendance. Test taking was a piece of cake. I guess I had a great memory because the test would answer it self. I really was not the friend type. I would meet other kids but to really call them friends they would have to prove that they were worthy of my friendship. I was not a spoiled brat but I did consider myself an intelligent kid and would only socialize, as far as making friends, with other good students. I did manage to make a few friends of which many disappeared in the transition of elementary school to middle school and then from middle school to high school. There was one person that stayed through the years. His name is Esteban "Barney". That nickname stuck with him his entire school career. We called him "Barney" because he would always be smiling with a great smile that looked just like Barney the dinosaur. After graduation I lost track of him. The last thing I knew of him was that he worked at Pizza Hut while attending school full time. Barney was an active runner; as a matter of fact in high school he holds records for the cross country team as well as for the track team.

One rainy afternoon I was driving by a local Pizza Hut since I had been on the road for quite some time I really needed to use the restroom So, I stopped to use the restroom. So I walked in and there he was, standing by the cash register. "Barney?" I said. He turned around and said, "Shhhhhhhhhhh". I guess he was trying to loose the old nick name. We spoke for about half an hour. Everything seemed to be going his way. He was doing well in school. He was really nervous because he was going to be running a marathon soon. I wished him the best of luck and hoped to see him soon. Pizza Hut got somewhat busy and Esteban had to work, so I used the restroom and then left.

Esteban was not my only friend. In middle school I met Carlos. Carlos is from Argentina and we used to tell everybody that we were twins. You see his birthday is on March 30 and mine is on March 31st. we have calculated that with the time zone change he is only minutes older than me. Carlos is a genius. Technically he can take a computer apart and rebuild it and make it work better than before. Carlos is a big muscular guy. He was on the school's swim team and water polo. He is a funny guy who can figure out almost any word problem no matter what the subject may be. In high school we had math and physics together. If we were in a class together I knew that I can count on him for group projects. We both loved similar subjects in school but we are so different at heart. He is the talkative and friend making type. While as you know I am the quiet one. Carlos loved to read sci-fi books, while I don't like to read for pleasure.

He is a Star Wars maniac, while I just like to watch the movies. Further more; we are both really good at playing strategic board games like checkers and chess. A chess game may take us several hours to declare a winner. However, most time it ends up as a stalemate. After high school Carlos went to a technology school while I went of to Cal State Fullerton. Soon after starting college I lost track of him, but luckily our destinies crossed. We now keep in touch.

As my working career kicked off I met several new people at work. I was working for Bank of America when I met Monica. Monica was also a student at Cal State Fullerton. I never saw her there but I believed her. We were both studying business administration, so I knew that she would be able to help me understand topics from class if I did not understand. Monica is a pretty and intelligent girl. She is very out going and also very cheerful. Her best friend also worked for the bank. Her name is Lizbet, but we all called her Betty because of her obsession with Betty Boob. Betty is a very nice girl who worked as a merchant teller. By the way Monica worked in new accounts. I got along great with every one at the bank. I loved to be at work because everyday there was something going on that made all of us happy. I think that we just loved to be around each other. For Valentines Day I gave a beautiful red rose to all of the ladies.

These girls were not just good friends but also great people you can talk to about personal problems knowing that your conversion would stay a secret. I do not know what the girls saw in me but I looked like I was the number one source to discuss their problems. I would be a rich man if I would have charge for listening to them. It was not just a few girls that would talk to me but all my co-workers. No matter what their problem was I was the first one to find out. I did not talk about my problem to anybody but Ana. Ana was one of the girls that I enjoyed talking too. She was a good friend. No matter what my problem was she was always there to listen and to help me. As you know I also met my first love at the bank. None of the girls that I worked with liked her. They told me that she had a bad attitude with them and that she always looked mad. Furthermore, before Jessica I did not know the meaning of music. I didn't pay any attention to what they said. I was happy with her. Jessica taught me how to dance and she introduced me to music. Before her the only thing I was into was school. She made me realize that there is more to life than just school.

All the girls at the bank were beautiful pieces of art, but only one had my complete attention. Her name is Jessica, no not my girlfriend of the time, a different Jessica and she is from Texas. Jessica has a twin sister, Vanessa that also worked for Bank of America but at another location. Jessica had beautiful soft hair that reached the soft skin of her shoulders. She also attended Cal State Fullerton and was studying business administration. I had a big crush on her, but I was too chicken to express my feelings. Plus I knew that she had a boyfriend and I was not single. For her birthday I gave her a dozen roses. Jessica has a pair of brilliant eyes and a pair of lips that would drive me crazy. Unfortunately I left a few months after she arrived. However, I did enjoy all the time that I spent working with her.

After a couple of years of not knowing what happened to her our roads crossed again. As you know I worked for Orange County Credit Union. Now more attractive than before she still drove me wild when I saw her. We have had lunch together a couple of times, you know she ate her lunch and I ate my lunch we just happened to bump into each other in the lunch room. After talking for a few minutes I found out that she is still with her boyfriend and very happy, but this time I was single. She is almost done with school, and can't wait to put her knowledge to work. I told her about all of the bumps that I have driven thru and how hard it has been to get back on my feet. For a moment her face turned into sadness, she looked down and then raised her head and said to me that knowing me she knew I would not give up.

Jessica was not the only person that I have bumped into at the Orange County Credit Union. I also had the opportunity to speak with Monica. She seems to be doing extremely well. After I transferred from Bank of America to Orange County Teachers FCU, an ex co-worker made the same move. Her name was Jessica, this was a different Jessica, and she was working for the Fountain Valley branch. It was unfortunate that we did not get to work at the same branch. I was located at the Santa Ana location After Jessica came to OCTFCU Elizabeth, Liz, came over as well. Fortunately,

Liz worked with me at the Santa Ana location. It was like the old days at Bank of America, fun and entertaining. Liz is a very cheerful and funny girl.

Although most of my friends I met at work. Teresa Duong or Teresa Ung like I like to call her is one of my best friends. Teresa was my trainer while I was in my ROP internship back in the day. She worked at the Mainplace mall location where I took my internship at. Like you know I was hired at 16 and worked at the Santa Ana office. Soon after I began my career Teresa was promoted to supervisor and was transferred to the Santa Ana office. Teresa is of Vietnamese culture, and she is very cool. She is still at Bank of America and attending school full time. I like to make fun of her because being Asian she is not the best of students. Not that I have something against Asians it is just that all of the Asians I have dealt with are very smart.

Teresa and I have always been in touch. She calls once in while to see how I am doing, and I call her to find out if she is still alive. You see she has a violent boyfriend and she worries me. I do not know why she is still with him but I guess its love. She always tells me that he has change, and I believe her because Teresa is the kind of person who speaks nothing but the truth. She is also the type of woman that you do not want to mess with. Just the look on her face is scary if she is mad. I cannot imagine it upset and angry at the same time. I am the only one who called her crouching tiger hidden dragon.

Most of my friends or acquaintances come from the work force.

Just recently I bumped eye contact with one of my basketball buddies from high school. His name is Eric and we bumped into each other at the gym where he worked for a very short time. I got his phone number and he got mine. At first he did not know that I was sick but then found out after I told him that I would not be able to play ball with the rest of the guys. We talk every now and then and usually hang out on Tuesday nights. Since he has kept in touch with some of the guys I got to see how Dan and Hanh were doing. Dan and Eric worked as security officers for a community in the city. Hanh had just gotten his Associates Degree and was now looking for a job. Like I mentioned we usually hang out on

Tuesday nights. We usually play pool or just hang out and play cards.

I am not really in communication with anybody simply because I do not like to bother anybody with my problems. I am the type of person that will keep everything inside locked up in a small chest that is hidden in the darkest spot of my heart. The only true friend that knows me inside out is Magda, and I know her better than anybody else. The way we met was really an adventure. That is why I believe that we are meant for each other. Even though, she is miles away I know that one day she will return and hopefully we will get back together. Magda is the only person that has seen me cry and the only person that I have shared my feelings with. You can call me woos, but I don't care simply because a good cry is good every once in a while. I do miss her, spiritually and physically. I miss talking to her and spending time with each other.

I may know several people but only one is a true friend. There is only one who I can trust. The one I can love and the one who I can laugh with. Otherwise, I am a lonely soul wondering the earth in search for the one who makes me whole.

Sidelines

As I mentioned earlier physical activities is one of my strongest weaknesses. Other than basketball I really sucked at everything else. I was not in the best of shape. I was pretty heavy and most of it was baby fat. As a freshman in high school I probably was about 5ft. 8 inches tall and weighted around 200lbs. In PE class, physical education, I was always the last person picked on a team. Whether we were playing soccer, volleyball, baseball or any other team sport I was always the last one picked. However, when the sport was basketball I was among the first ones to be picked. Everybody knew that basketball was my sport.

I hated running around the track. I got tired really quick and always finished among the last group. I hated PE class. Being the last one picked for a team always hurt and it damaged my self steam. It hurt but the only thing I was able to do was to try my best and forget what every one else thought.

I loved to play basketball. I remember that I used to get to school an hour or so before class so that I would be able to play ball. I used to take my basketball with me every morning. Most of the time other students showed up and we got ourselves a full court game going. I loved to shoot the ball from the three point line. However my game was in the post. I didn't care if you were bigger or taller than me. In the post I was the one in control. When it came to playing defense I loved to defend the ball handler. I had quick hands and there was nobody in the court that was able to dribble pass me.

I had a really good shot. I hardly missed. It didn't matter where I was shooting from, the ball always went in. Students told me that I should try out for the school team. My junior year the coach saw me one day and asked me to try out. Try outs were after school and I had to work, so I never tried out. Anyways, try outs were not just about basketball. It also involved getting in shape and like I mentioned earlier I hated PE.

My dad although in his middle age is still a good basketball player. He shoots about 80% from the field and probably shoots better than that from behind the arc. My dad and I used to spend Friday nights at the park. We would play for money and on a good night we would make almost $50.00. As my brother got older he would also come along with us. My brother can play. He has dribbles, hops, and a nice shot. His only problem back then was that he had butter fingers.

Anyways when all three of us played together we were unstoppable. I took care of the post. My brother handled the ball and my dad took care of the perimeter. Those days were great. I miss those times. Now I can't even dribble a basketball without loosing control. I can't run up and down the court and I definitely can't jump. I can still shoot the ball but it has to be from a short range. I hate not being in the game.

I have gone to the park several times and just watch the games going on from the side line. Every once in a while someone comes up to me and asks if I want to play. My heart jumps into action while I just sit there and say no thanks. I hate it because I really want to play. Multiple sclerosis has caused me to dribble out of bounce into the side line. I sit here waiting for my turn. I am tired of being in the side lines but I know that the game will one day be in my court.

The Multi-tasked

Growing up was difficult for me. Not only did my parents request good grades in school but also to set a prime example for my brothers to follow. School was not difficult at all. After kinder garden I began to discover my skills in the arts of doing something while doing something else.

School was kind of easy for me. All that I needed to do was show up for class, and my brain just recorded what the teacher said, even if I was doing something else. Being in class was easy because my parents took me to school every day. Like you know I received the perfect attendance award every year. The hardest thing for me was homework. I hated it and I never did it at home. I always did homework in class. Not the class where it was due, but in class. I usually did my physics homework in English class and I usually did my pre-calculus homework in history class. If I had history homework I usually did it in home room. If I had any other homework I would do it in pre-calculus class. I never liked homework but unfortunately the only homework I did at home was English homework because it usually involved reading or writing an essay.

I do not know how I did it. I guess it was just a gift or talent that I possessed. It was something very cool, because when it came to test time I never had to prepare for it. That is right. I never studied for a test, and when it came to the actual test: it just answered it self. What I mean is that the answers came to mind as I read the question or problem. Sometimes all I had to do was think about the problem and I was able to hear the teacher talk about the solution in my head. It is really strange but if I think about it I can replay a conversation in my head. I never failed a test, and I do not recall a test score under 85%. The only test I remember studying for where my SAT's. I received an average score of 1280. I was happy with my score.

I guess being a good listener helped with this talent. I never felt stressed or worried about an upcoming test. I knew that I had been in class and had listened to everything the teacher said. I knew that when it was test time I would remember everything that had been taught in class and homework assignments. Furthermore, I believe that if I was to retake the same test today I'm certain that I would still receive a similar score if not better.

Another thing that I was capable of doing was talking about something while thinking about something completely different. For example there were times when I was doing my math homework and the history teacher would ask me something in reference to the class topic. I would have no problem answering the question even if I was dealing with polynomials or math formulas. I do not know how I did it. I just did.

It may sound strange or amazing but believe it or not; it is true. I have learned that multitasking is a rare reason for M.S. But unfortunately it looks like the skills I developed growing up had its consequences. Consequences that I am know dealing with. Although, there are many reasons for developing multiple sclerosis, I think that multitasking is the reason why I have M.S.

The Human Pincushion

Kenishowa….In Japanese it means a new day. It is definitely a new day in my life, especially with a new reason to live. Magda is still miles away from my heart but it feels like she is still with me everywhere I go. I have not forgotten about Magda, I have just found an alternative to dealing with the M.S. I have found relaxation through acupuncture, and hope that my numbness for once will disappear.

My dad has been suffering from neck pain for the past couple of days. A good friend of his referred him to the South Baylo University of Acupuncture and Herbal Medicine. After a couple of treatments my dad felt better, and it was at that point that he asked if they treated M.S. The answer was yes, and before you knew it I became a patient. The first consultation was free but then it would be $25.00 per consultation plus the cost of herbs. However, since I still had my student I.D from Cal State Fullerton my consultation cost was only $7.00.

It was at the clinic that I have pick up a little bit of Japanese, Korean, and even some Chinese. It is at this clinic that I have meet great people. The doctors have told me that they have had a great success with their other M.S. patients. They also told me not to expect quick results because they tell me that it usually takes anywhere from six months to a year before their patients notice changes. The first time I attended the clinic I was seen by Dr. Yu. Dr. Yu is an old woman with a mysterious look in her black eyes. Her English is not perfect but understandable. She told me that she actually had her PHD in dealing with M.S. and of course I got to see the diploma. After many years as director of the clinic she has pass down her thrown to an ex-student of hers Dr. Lien.

I have to mention that when I first walked into the clinic I was scare of the pain the needles may cause me. With my skin still being hypersensitive the pain I may feel terrified me. Dr. Skinner did this test on me to find out how severe the hypersensitivity was. She would test me by poking me with a fine needle and she would ask me to describe how it felt, whether it was extremely sharp, sharp, or dull. I swear that at my worst stage that fine needle would feel like a stab from a really sharp knife. I knew that my hypersensitivity had improved, but I still shook in my boots with fear. After meeting Dr. Yu we came up with a great schedule for my treatment. I would see Dr. Yu on Tuesday evenings and Dr. Lien on Thursday evenings. Dr. Yu acupunctures my spinal cord and then followed it up with a deep tissue massage. Dr. Lien did acupuncture on my arms and legs. Since this is a University you are first seen by interns. They take your vitals ask you questions and then the doctor will come in and see you. The doctor decides what points to assign and interns then acupuncture you.

For a man with very sensitive skin let me tell you that it is not painful at all. Unless you get kidney one assigned to you. Kidney one is a point located right in the center of your foot. The point is not really painful; the insertion of the needle is like a small poke. What hurts is the stimulation of the needle, when they turn the needle.

I don't always get the same interns but I think that I have met all of them. Most interns love to treat me because no matter what doctor is seeing me I always get about 30 different points. I am a target practice for the interns. I don't worry because they are always under supervision. The needles stay in you for about 15 minutes. Although I look like a human pincushion I find it very relaxing.

I know most of the interns by name, even though their names are hard to pronounce I make the effort. One name I know how to pronounce is Lawrence. Lawrence sees me almost on every single one of my visits. He is a very cool guy and I really trust him with the acupuncture. I know he is a student but he is a good one to be dealing with. Gin Ju is another good intern. Everybody calls her Ginger because of the spelling similarity and easier pronunciation. Her name means "Pearl" in English and I swear that the shine in her eyes speak for her. I told her once that I just loved her bright eyes and from that moment on she would get really shy around me. She turned red in a hurry with me not even having to say a word.

It has only been about a month that I have been receiving this acupuncture treatment but I feel optimistic about the results that can result from this. I have not yet notice any changes but I do feel more relaxed then before. I think the relaxation comes from the herbs that I have been taking. Hopefully the relaxation will lead to my numbness improving.

My Fear

The fact of the matter is that I am not the same Edwin I once was. I fear what tomorrow will bring. I fear not knowing if it is really coming. We walk our path in destiny and I fear what this illness can do to me. I hate not being able to do what the old Edwin did. I am scared of what is to come.

I hate the fact that I can no longer enjoy the things that I used to do. The memories of me having a good time hurt. It is pain like no other. I can't breathe and it hurts to watch others enjoy life. The fact that I can no longer go out and play basketball is killing me. I miss shooting around with my dad. I miss dribble ling the ball up and down the court.

I hate the fact that I can't dance. Although I did not dance much I was good, and I hate the fact that I get tired really fast. My legs feel like hot rubber and I hate it. I hate feeling mentally capable of doing things and not being capable of such thing. Maybe I try too hard but I hate thinking that I can do anything.

I fear that the day when I can do anything will never come. I miss the little things. The things I did not do much off. Things like roller blade or riding a bike. With my balance problems that appears to be nothing more than a dream. I hate the fact that I cannot run in the rain. I fear that I will never be able to do these things. I fear that I won't be able to teach my son or daughter how to ride a bike. I fear not being able to have fun with them. I fear the fact that I will not be able to play ball with my children

I fear that I won't be able to overcome this bump on the road.

I fear the fact that I am different. My darkest fear is of what multiple sclerosis can do to me. I fear not being able to do the things that I do now. I am scare because I know that an exacerbation, a relapse, can happen at any time and there is nothing I can do to avoid it. I fear that I may not be able to stand under my own power. I am scared that I may be in a wheel chair tomorrow. I fear being in a vegetative state.

I fear loosing my freedom. I hate the fact that I know what can happen. Knowledge is making me fear my fears.

The Face in the Mirror

With everything happening so fast and with all the ups and downs that my life has been through I had forgotten about the real world. The face in the mirror was a familiar one. It was definitely my face but it certainly was not me in the picture. My face was the same but I was now looking at a new man.

My eyes were different. The sparkle in the eyes that I had once possessed was no longer there. The sincerity in my eyes was also gone and unfortunately I knew it was gone for good. I now have a deep mysterious look that opens the window to a dark place, a dark place that I did not dare to explore. The Edwin that I once knew was no more. The joy that once ran through my vanes had vanished.

I knew a new Edwin had been born from all the suffering that I had endured. The kindness that I once processed is no longer the same. Now I look at the outcome for me before helping somebody. Everything has to be to my advantage. I think that after being away from the real world for so long I need to catch up with everybody else. I know that this new feeling is not right but unfortunately I do not see my self changing that characteristic for a good time or until a feel ahead of everybody else.

The truth is that I am not happy with myself. I know that I have fought time and time again to prove to myself that I can do it. Unfortunately the smile in the mirror is a fake one. It is a duplicate of the smile that I once enjoyed. A fake smile hoping it tricks people into believing that I am happy. I do not want people's pity or help, so I force myself to show everybody else that I am okay.

I do not know myself anymore and I know that one day I will be able to see the monster that I have become. The face in the mirror will no longer be mine but of the scary monster I would have become.

I have gone through many changes; one for example is that I am huge and over weight. My clothes tightly fit and my shoes are too big. My feet have shrunk a bit and the sad part was that it was not the only thing that had shrunk. My confidence level in regards to satisfying a woman has rapidly diminished but as time went by I learned that I was still the stallion I once was. Fire ran through my vanes when I was intimate, and it made me feel real god. My body shakes a bit and it is kind of hard to hide. I guess the shaking helped in my sex life, but I did not like it one bit. My balance is not perfect and it is very difficult to walk at a fast pace, or in a straight line. Furthermore, it is impossible to even try running. Now that I cannot run I feel the desire to run. I feel like a trapped hare. Not being able to run free is painful. My body continues to be numb, especially my hands and feet. The numbness in my feet does not worry me as much as the numbness in my hands. There are times when the numbness in my feet and legs feels strange. My legs feel weird. They feel as if I had spilled soda on myself. "You know" that sticky feeling that just won't go away. Sometimes every thing feels uncomfortable. I am happy as long as I can walk, but the numbness in my hands make it very difficult to complete simple duties. Simple tasks such as brushing my teeth or eating, and typing is very difficult if not almost impossible. The numbness has decreased the sensibility in my hands making them feel almost stiff and heavy. Everything I touch feels rough like sand paper. Warm water feels too hot and cold water feels like ice water. Now I get cold really easily.

The best way of describing the way my hands feel is the way your hand feels when you fall at sleep on your hand, and blood does not circulate to your hand. It is an ugly feeling that unfortunately I have to deal with 24 hours a day, seven days a week. Emotionally I feel very vulnerable and scared. I hide my emotions and appear not to be damaged or scared at all. I do not show my emotions. I seem to hide everything with the smile in the mirror. Whether I am having difficulties controlling my symptoms or I am just having a bad day. A friendly smile is always on my face.

The only thing that really has not change is my confidence. I still posses an overachieving attitude. I strive to be all that I can be. I have a positive mentality. I want to touch the clouds and then reach for the stars. I believe that if you want something you must earn it no matter how hard you may have to strive. I still posses the fighting attitude that has help me overcome my disabilities. I believe that a "push" will get you anywhere except thru a door that says "pull". I force myself to believe that if I am incapable of doing something today; I will be able to do it tomorrow, and if not tomorrow then the day after. I have matured a lot, and according to people that knew the follower that I once was. They now say that a new leader has emerged. The few friends that I have know that I will stop at nothing until I am driving on the right road. Even though, I am still struggling with most of my symptoms I will not be happy until I overcome this tall bump.

I hope that once the road is plain for me the Edwin that hides in the darkest part of my heart will once again emerge, and once again the face in the mirror will be mine. I just need to remember that I am not the man underneath the mask but that only my actions define who I am. The face in the mirror will be mine and I will be the one in control.

Darkness

Many weeks have now flown by since my last entry. The summer is now gone and cold winds have now emerge. Magda is still gone and frankly I feel like her childhood doll, untouched and forgotten. Unfortunately, we only talk when I call her. She does not call to say hi, or to see how I am doing. I really miss her, so much that it hurts not to hear from her. She tells me she loves me, but I just ignore it. I tell her to prove it but she just goes cold. I cannot stand feeling like a worn out doll and unfortunately, it has caused the flame that once burned between us to become nothing more than a bursting spark.

It is late October 2004 and I am tired of feeling forgotten. I can not say that I do not love her because I do, maybe even more than yesterday. I desire her more than ever. I dream of her at night and I think of her every minute of my life. Although it hurts very much I called her yesterday and ended the adventure that we had lived. She took it well; I guess she was expecting it. She got upset as I explain that I could no longer continue feeling forgotten. She sounded like she was just about to burst into tears and she then hung up. I also told her that I never meant to hurt her but unfortunately our lives were not meant for each other at that time.

The M.S. appears to be under control. I have know been attending my acupuncture therapy for a couple of months. Even though, I have not experience any dramatic changes, I am optimistic. Doctors tell me that it will take some time to see changes. The fear of pain, which I once had, has completely banished since I have now experience no discomfort ness.

Since we are now in October, the weather is no longer an allied but an enemy. My hands feel number than before almost stiff. Movement is still good but more difficult than before. My feet are beginning to feel number than usual: especially my left foot. I would think that with the colder weather my eye sight would improve because I did not have to worry about the daylight brightness.

Unfortunately, the cold weather has not help. For being a warm person I have often feel cold. So cold that my feet feel like ice at some points. My feet feel so frozen that it sometimes alters the way I walk. It has been raining for the past couple of days and the forecast says that even more rain is coming this way. The rain makes it very difficult to focus, especially if I am driving. When it rains everybody drives with their lights on. Since it is usually dark when it rains the light and the falling water hurt my eyes. For my safety and the safety of others I avoid driving anywhere but work and my home.

This cold weather makes me think about Magda even more frequent. I miss keeping her warm since she is the type of person that gets cold by just eating ice cream. I miss talking with her, but now more than ever I have to try to forget.

I have tried my best not to call her but I just can't go anther day with out hearing her beautiful, soft angel voice. It was Thanksgiving Day evening. I had just finished eating with the family. I called her hoping that she wanted to hear from me. Luckily, she was the one who picked up. I started by saying hello and asking her how she was doing. She said fine and asked how I was doing. I responded by saying "I am doing okay, but I feel like something great is missing." She laughed a little and said "Well why don't you look for it." We had a conversation going. I told her that I missed her and that everyday without her became more painful. She said she missed me too and that only time would tell if our roads would cross again. We talked for about an hour before I realized that in Mexico it was almost midnight. I told her that I did not want to keep her up and wished her a good night.

It felt good talking to her, so good that I began to regret what I had done to her. Since then it has become easier to not think about her so much but I still miss her, maybe more than before.

There was one night when I really felt good, so good that I went dancing. I went to Cuban Pete's, a small Cuban restaurant and night club located close to Disneyland. They were playing great music. I love the tropical rhythm, especially salsa. Before I was diagnosed I had taken salsa lessons and used to dance with some of the girls from Bank of America. They said I was really good, but I did not know if it was true. It was not hard to find the rhythm seating down. My head was bobbling, my feet were tapping, but when I got on my feet it all changed. I felt like a drunken man trying to stay on his feet. My legs felt as if they could have collapse at any time. It was horrible I was struggle ling very much to stay on my feet. My legs felt like hot rubber. That night I got to dance with a couple of girls but they told me that I felt really stiff and to relax. I felt that if I would have relaxed I would have fallen down, like an unstoppable mud slide. One of them even abandoned me in the middle of the dance floor. It hurt, it really hurt. Just when I thought that for a minute I would not have to worry about anything and just have some fun. I felt like the world had collapse on me. I have tried other ways of distracting myself, like hanging out more with a couple of old buddies. Furthermore, the gym has become my second life. If I am not home or at work you can bet that you can find me at the gym.

During the time that Magda has been away I have tone up and have lost about 30 lbs. I feel in great shape even though the numbness in my feet has gotten worse. After a couple of years of not being able to loose any weight I finally got too. Dr. Skinner said that I had been unable to loose weight because the drugs, steroids, were still in my system even though I had been off of them for a year. At one point I was weighing in at 255lbs. I am now at 220lb, and looking forward to loosing more weight.

Christmas soon came about and my feelings towards Magda grew. I missed her more than ever before. I desired her more than before. I wanted to hold her real bad but I knew she was out of the reach of my finger tips. I called her with the excuse of wishing her a Merry Christmas and a Happy New Year. I missed her like the land misses the sun during the night time. The light that once glowed in my heart had left with her departure living nothing more than darkness.

Magda was my world; she was the only thing that mattered. Most importantly she was my inspiration. She was my daylight, she was the sun that brightened my heart and with her departure she took everything with her; leaving darkness.

Time Out

I hope 2005 brings me better luck in this sick game of life. I start the year behind everybody else. January has been a very rainy month that has brought down bad luck for people in the hills. The rain has been so bad that houses have tumble down the muddy hills. Anaheim Hills has had some houses demolished to prevent damage to other houses. Unfortunately, the people of La Conchita were not so lucky. A mud slide destroyed several houses that slid down the hills and buried several lives. There were over ten deaths reported.

In my case, I was glad that I did not suffer as much as those people did. In Asia there was a tsunami that hit the coast killing thousands of people. There was no specific count because dead bodies continued to appear in the beach every day. It was devastating to start the year with so many lives being lost.

In my case the rain prevented me from driving anywhere other than work and the gym. I did not even go to the gym as usual due to the fear of hurting someone or myself. My feet are beginning to feel number than usual, and my skin feels a bit more sensitive. However, I can still manage to do everyday activities with no difficulties. My eye sight is not all that great but it has not gotten worst than before. I can still see fine as long as I wear my shades and as long as the lights are turned down. I fear having a relapse. I have recently started feeling some new symptoms. There are times when my face feels numb. It tingles and my face feels deformed. Sometimes it feels difficult to open my mouth. That is not the only new symptom; sometimes my tongue feels like it is tangled up in my throat. Although in my head I sound normal when I tape recorded myself I realized that my speech is impaired. I have also felt strange at times. It feels like all my movements are in slow motion. There are also times when everything seems like its spinning. Luckily it only lasts for a few seconds. Another new symptom is strange. Sometimes when I walk I get these spasms. My body feels the need to stretch my leg muscles while I am walking causing me to look like Bambi giving his first steps. It is weird and I do not know how to avoid the spasms. There is nothing that can put me down. My attitude is good and I believe that as long as I "push" I will be okay. I believe that it is not impossible to reach the untouchable.

My Last Hope

It is mid February 2005. My symptoms appear to be under control but still make simple tasks somewhat difficult. I have realized that I am not like I used to be. I am a new person, a new person that I have to learn to love. I have to learn how to like my self because only by doing so I will be able to be happy, and if the mind is happy the body is happy.

The numbness in my body has not disappeared but I try not to think about it hoping that my mind will forget. My hands feel stiff but I do not let that stop me from doing anything. My eye sight is not all that great. It is actually pretty bad. So, bad that driving is dangerous. I am hoping to see an ophthalmologist soon.

I do not seem to be able to stop thinking about Magda lately. I still miss her with all my heart. I still call her every once in a while. The last time that I spoke with her she told me that we would spend her birthday together. I knew it was a lie but my heart was filled with joy. I don't understand why love is this way. We know the truth, yet the mind follows the heart.

A Push

I do not say this much but I truly believe that "A push can get you anywhere. It can teach you many things, but the only thing it can't do is get you thru a door that says pull." In my quote, I believe the word push means effort. It mainly states that as long as you try you will achieve. There is a fighter in me that will not give up and a warrior in my soul that will not give in to disappointment. I think that no matter what you have, no matter what you are suffering from your attitude is the way out of those dark places.

I have done it before and I believe that every body with the heart can do it. Do not give up, do not be a quitter. Do not be like those people who aim at nothing and always succeed. Set your goals high, and fight. Do not aim at nothing because I will guarantee that you will get there. I have been at a point so low that I wished that I no longer woke up from a night sleep. I have been so depressed that life meant nothing to me. Now look at me; I am back on my feet and little by little accomplishing new things. Sure, I have had my ups and downs but I am always pushing on the worst of my days.

February is now coming to an end and the rain has finally calmed down. My symptoms have gotten worse but I am pushing to continue my life style. My feet are now completely stiff and my skin is more hypersensitive than before. I can still wear my regular clothes, but it is beginning to feel uncomfortable from the waist down. My sight remains the same but I try to avoid the bright sunny days. My gym routine is becoming a bit difficult. I am getting tired quicker and my leg strength is decreasing. I can still walk fine but a limp is beginning to emerge.

I am focusing on staying in shape to work. I am exercising every chance I get and watching closely what I eat. Even with my extra efforts March is becoming a challenge. It is now early March, and my walking has gotten worse. I am limping more than before but I am still doing my best to hide it and look normal as much as possible. My hands feel number than usual and the stiff feeling is beginning to emerge. Flexibility in my hands is still good but not as good as it has been. My tremor problems are the only thing that the acupuncture has taken care of. I do not shake as much as I used too and I am happy for that. I am not getting as much rest I used too because it is becoming difficult to fall at sleep. When I get up in the mornings I feel very tired and weak. Further more, my muscles ache and concentrating at work is difficult. I feel fatigued all the time and being at the gym is only a dream.

It has gotten so bad that hiding the fatigue has become impossible. Like I have mentioned earlier I hide my feelings because I do not need anybodies pity. It bugs me to know that someone is worrying for me and I do not want that even for my parents. I've been feeling exhausted almost daily and have scheduled an appointment with Dr. Skinner.

The week before my birthday I got to see Dr. Skinner. She tells me that she sees me in bad shape. She asked me for my symptoms. I responded by saying, "Same oh same oh, just worse than usual." She did a strength test on me were she discovered that I was weaker than the last time she saw me. Her tests consist of trying to maintain my ground while she tries to move me. For example, she has me lift my leg as she tries to bring it down. The last time that I saw her she was unable to bring my legs down or even move them an inch. This was not the case this time. Even though, it took her effort she had no problem moving my legs down.

I admitted, I was in bad shape but I did not want to be taken off of work like she suggested. Not wanting to be in the disability situation again, I begged asking her to let me continue working. We discussed the issue and luckily for me she changed her mind. She placed me on a limited work order. I would now be able to work daily, but only for a maximum of 5 hours per day.

My new schedule at work was now 10 a.m. to 3 p.m. it was very relaxing at first but when I got to see my paycheck I realized that I would not be able to keep the same life style. Since I was now working at 10 a.m. I was able to get more sleep. Soon I began to feel less tired, and was able to save energy for the gym. Since, my work day ended early in the afternoon I was able to get more rest. Further more, I began to feel better as well as stronger.

After a full month of restricted work hours I got to see Dr. Skinner for a follow up. Sure, I was in better shape than my previous visit with her, but still she did not remove the work hour restriction. Instead she increased it to a six hour work day maximum. I asked Dr. Skinner to refer me to the ophthalmology department because for the past few weeks I have been suffering from vision problems. Not only am I having vision problems but my eyes itch and are very red. I bought some over the counter eye drops but they do not seem to work at all.

The following day I got to see the ophthalmologist. Dr. Smith. He is a very nice doctor who prescribed me some eye drops that helped eliminate the itch and redness in my eyes. He took the time to ask me some questions in regards to the medication that I was taking. He asked me several questions to how my sight has been since my diagnoses. I told him that for a moment I was almost completely blind and that now my eyes are extremely sensitive to the light. I told him that the other ophthalmologist had just recommended me to wear dark shades but none of them recommended glasses. I told him that I need help with my eye sight because I have problems focusing. I told him that if I can get use to the light surrounding me I can read the newspaper. When it came to taking the eye exam; I found it very hard to see the letters on the board. My score was horrible it made my previous score of 17/20 look great. My over all score was 20/70 in my left eye and 20/400 in my right eye. After knowing what I scored you must think I am blind. To tell you the truth my shades help me out a lot.

My shades block out enough sunlight from my eyes that makes driving dangerous but possible. Sometimes I may not be able to distinguish the color of the vehicle in front but at least I can see it. Sometimes I cannot see what color the light is in so I just go with traffic. I think that I have run over 2 red lights. Two close calls because I saw the light turn from orange to red as I crossed. Sometimes I can make out the color signal and that is great but sometimes I notice the light color too late and I have to slam on my brakes or step on the gas. Even though, I admit needing help with my eye sight, doctors do not think I need glasses. Hopefully now I will have glasses prescribed to me, and my sight problem would be the least of my problems.

Dr. Smith prescribed me three infusions of Solimedrole. If you recall, I have had this treatment before. Although, this time I was taking it to improve my eye sight: the side effects would be the same. I had to ask for some time off of work so that I would be able to attend the infusion. Luckily, the infusion center was able to schedule me for three consecutive visits. I felt stronger after every visit, but unfortunately my eye sight did not appear to have improved. My legs were stronger and even some of the numbness has improved. The hypersensitivity I had been feeling has decreased. Unfortunately, the concerns about my vision remain the same.

A couple of weeks after the infusions I got to see Dr. Smith for a follow up. Even though, I have felt no difference in my eyes sight the tests proved me wrong. After taking the vision exam he told me that my vision was now at 20/50. You might think that it was a big improvement, but to be honest; it was only an improvement on paper. I was still dealing with the same problems and driving was still dangerous. I asked Dr. Smith to prescribe me glasses but instead he referred me to an optometrist.

I got to see the optometrist two days later, but unfortunately he was not able to prescribe me glasses because by that time my vision had changed. After taking another vision test it was revealed that my vision was now worse than when I saw Dr. Smith. The optometrist asked me if my vision changed frequently. I told him that it varies from day to day and that it depended on the weather. He asked me in what type of weather was my vision at its best. I told him that on cloudy and cool days. He suggested that I consider moving up north to a colder state. I saw him again two days later and my vision test score was different. So, with my eye sight changing so frequently he was not able to prescribe any type of glasses. So, I continue driving hoping that I did not hurt anyone.

I was really beginning to feel tired of the same routine and having to be at work at the time that I was scheduled. The people I was working with were great but I was getting tired of following the same routine day after day. After thinking of what I really wanted for weeks I decided to leave OCCU and work on my own through Primerica financial services. I had been involved with Primerica for almost the same amount of time that I was at OCCU but had not really done business with them because the pay was only commission based. So on July 2005 I began to explore new grounds as my own boss. My success depends on me and you can bet that I will push to my limits.

Heartbroken

The last time that I spoke with Magda she had promised me that we were going to spend her birthday together. Even though I knew she wasn't telling the truth my heart felt warm with joy and happiness. Her birthday was on July 6, but she was a no show. I called her to wish her a happy birthday but she was not home. I tried a couple other times but her sister always told me that she wasn't home.

I was really hoping to see her soon. It felt like my last chance to save our love had shatter. Unfortunately, I have not tried to speak with her since.

I am starting to realize that maybe she doesn't want to return and that all that we lived was a complete lie. Who knows? Only tomorrow will tell if our paths will cross again and if anything is going to happen between us. But for now it is best I don't call her and try to forget.

So I stand alone hoping that my new life as my own boss goes well.

Latin Tom Cruise

During my time at Orange County Credit Union I met great new people. Really cool people, really fun people like Alfredo and Joanna. I started working for OCCU mid June of 2004. As of July of 2005 I was no longer employed by them but by myself. Anyways, the time I spent there was great.

Like I mentioned I had a couple of re-acquaintances while at OCCU but most importantly I got to meet new people. At first I thought that I would not fit in because everybody looked so serious, but once they had a piece of me the tension was broken.

I met Armando," the Cuban Dance Machine". Armando was really cool not only was he great assisting members but fun and entertaining with all of the team. We went out as a group once and that night was one for the books. We went to Cuban Petes a nice restaurant/nightclub located behind Disneyland. We laughed, drank some nice Caribbean drinks, and danced the night away. That was when we found out why they called him "the Cuban dance machine".

Another great person was Fabby, Fabby worked in the account services department. Fabby was the one I mostly bugged with problems. Since she loves being the center of attention; I figured that she would have all the answers. She wanted so much attention that when I told her that I was writing a book she demanded a full chapter just on her. Telling her about my book was a big mistake because every day she would ask if I was done with her chapter. She was cool don't get me wrong but sometimes it felt like a routine when I saw her.

Let me tell you about my home boy John. John was one of the first person's that I made contact with. Our desks were next to each other so I had to talk to him. He only worked part time and attended school full time. John is the type of guy that would make you think "he goes to school". John is a smart guy, but even a funnier man. It was hilarious when he worked because he would tell some members that his name was John and would tell others that he was Miles. It was funny because we would sit there and listen to how at the end of his conversation by stating a different name to the caller.

The girls were great, Joanna, Nancy Jeana, Gaby, Imy, Juliana, Adriana, Estela, Nora, and Anne. Jeana and Gaby were in the management department so everything stayed professional. They were cool people don't get me wrong, but you do not want to say something that can affect the relationship at work. Imy always had to spell her name to the members. She would say, "Imy like Amy but with an I", it was funny because she would repeat it three or four times before the member finally understood what her name was. I did not interact much with Adriana, Anne, Estela, Nora or Juliana because their desks were out of reach. They were all cool girls.

Joanna and Nancy however sat behind me. We got to talk when it slowed down. Both of these girls are very pretty and have a great sense of humor. These were the girls that I was the closest too. Since I saw them every day they were more than just another person.

The person I really miss though is not one of the girls but my home boy Freddy. Alfredo had the same problem Imy did. They would always ask him how his name was spelled and he would answer by saying." it is Alfredo...... like the sauce". Freddy is Hispanic like myself so we bonded as friends fairly quick. Freddy was very cool because he understood my disabilities and always helped me without making it a big deal and that is very important to me because I do not like to be helped. Freddy is a funny man; he always, like myself, had a small prank up his sleeve. Freddy gave me the nickname "Latin Tom Cruise". Why? Who knows, but I am sure it has to do with what I wore every day. I always wore a nice suit with my cool shades and always walked in with my head raised up high like I owned the place.

My days at OCCU were definitely unforgettable, but with my eye sight really bothering me and making it very difficult to see the computer screen I decided to leave. For know I work on my own through Primerica financial services. Furthermore, I am planning on returning to school and getting a real estate license so that I sale homes down the line. Who knows what tomorrow will bring and I want to be prepare for what ever is thrown at me next.

The Healer

It is now August 2005; it has been a bit over three years that I have been living with M.S. They have been three hectic years but I am still here pushing. I have not given up because I know that I can beat this. I have lost the love of my love but I am not letting that sadness stop me. The hope for a cure is so big that I no longer feel the need to call Magda. I have found happiness within myself. I let the kid in me come out and play when ever he feels like coming out. Just yesterday I rolled down the biggest hill at the park and it felt great. I did not care what the people thought when they saw a 22 year old man in a business suit roll down the hill.

I have learned that the only way that I am going to be able to beat M.S is by being happy with me, no matter how different I may be. I push harder than ever so that I can prove to myself that I can still do the things I love.

Although, my symptoms have not improve I am keeping a positive attitude and not giving up because I know that I can be victorious.

My mom just got back from her homeland of El Salvador. She was there for two weeks visiting her brothers and sisters. Unfortunately, my cousin was killed during her stay there. While she was there she heard rumors of a healer, an old man who lived in the middle of no where. This proclaimed healer has cured many people from unbelievable illnesses. When my mom got back she convinced me of taking a trip down south to look for this man.

So, there I was on a plane to El Salvador the following week. The flight was about four and a half hours long, but it felt immortal since I was unable to sleep. The flight took place at night so the night felt like it was not coming to an end. My cousins picked me up at the airport and from there it was another two hours to get home. I stayed with my aunt and her grandsons.

The trip was great simply because I got to see my family, family that I had not seen in over 12 years. I learned that I had a great family. I bonded well with everyone especially with Glenda. Glenda is my cousin but after a couple of hour of meeting her she became something more. She became my confident, we talked about everything: her life, my love and my pains. She gave me great advice and told me to focus on what I want. Glenda is everything I look for in a woman. She is beautiful with a great sense of understanding, and most importantly very affectionate. I swear.... If she was not my cousin I would have fallen in love. She made me realize that if Magda really loved me she would not have leaved me in the first place. Glenda made me realize that I was living in a fairy tale and I had control of the outcome.

My feelings towards Magda changed. I still love her but I do not feel the need to call her anymore. Glenda made me realize that I have done so much without her and there is no reason for me to slow down and wait for her. I have realized that life is only a test for what is to come.

Father Renato, my cousin, took me to see this proclaimed healer. It took four hours to get to his house. When we got there he had about 10 people waiting to see him. I thought that everyone got individual consultations but I was wrong. He asked all of us to follow him into his bedroom. The room was very small, and was decorated with religious pictures on the walls. We sat down and he began his prayer for sanitation. Glenda was also with me. We were sitting together so whispering was possible. The healer was asking the lord for forgiveness and to please cure all the illnesses that were present when Glenda whispered," I am hungry". "Me too", I whispered back. We sat there listening to the old man while he continued asking god to take the illnesses as a sacrifice.

He then asked us to ask for forgiveness as he walked around the room placing his hand on his patient's heads. He really surprised me when he identified the illnesses that each one of us had. He placed his hand on our heads and asked the lord to take our symptoms with him.

When he finished asking for each one of us he asked us if we felt anything when he touched us. A couple of people said that they felt warmth, of course their was about 15 people in a small room, my aunt who was also there said that she felt like her feet were on ice. He asked me what I felt and I said "hunger", and he laughed. Then he asked Glenda and she said "nothing", which was the same thing I felt. Then we left and spoke no more of what we had experienced. Now it is time to wait and see if we are cure.

They say that this proclaimed healer has cured a couple of cancer patients but only time will tell if our illnesses will disappear.

In my opinion, this was all a joke. Sure, people have faith in this man, but all he does is fill your head with faith and hope. If you ask me, the cure to all illness is within us. If we believe that we are fine the body thinks that it is and by acts of miracles the illness disappears.

The cure to all of our problems is inside all of us. If we can be happy with ourselves we can accomplish a state of complete happiness, a state that I feel far from accomplishing. I feel great because I am happy with myself. I pay no attention to my symptoms I am just trying to be happy and pushing for more.

Faith will cure me because I believe that I am going to beat this rare disorder. I believe that I can do anything and as long as I believe I will be able to do anything that I want. This is exactly what I have always believed. If you remember I said that my motto was," if I cannot do it today I will be able to do it tomorrow and if not, then the day after".

Life is a sick game that has no shortcuts only daylight will tell us of what is to come. The hope to see daylight of the day when I am cured is what keeps me from giving up. It may take years but I know that the day will come.

A couple of days after seeing the healer I returned home re-energized and ready to continue my life. Since I have no job to return to, I will put myself to work by pushing for a better tomorrow.

The Cure

Recently, there has been talk about a man that the U.S. government is trying to sensor. His name is Kevin Trudeau and he is the author of *Natural Cures*. In his book he talks about how the cures to most disease and illnesses are being kept away from the public. He states that there are cures for many illnesses but we do not hear of them because the FDA would loose money. He states that the FDA would not be able to treat the illnesses so they would not be making any money. I agree with him completely because it just proves why there has not been a cure since the cure for polio.

In his book he gives what he has discovered to be the natural cures to relieve cancer, diabetes, and other illnesses. The cure for M.S. is not among the fifty diseases that he mentions but he does explain a diet that can help reduce the symptoms. This diet consists of eating only organic foods and walking for an hour every day. He suggests that I should bounce on a re-bounder for ten minutes everyday and sleep on a magnetic pad.

Believe it or not I have been doing my best at eating nothing but organic foods. I bought a re-bounder, a small trampoline, and jump on it every day. At first I was not able to do anything but bounce. However as time went by I began to jump. I am walking one hour everyday and in just two weeks I lost over 10 pounds. My balance has improved dramatically and most importantly I feel great. I am slimmer and trimmer. I have been able to burn more fat in my body. He suggested that I eat three apples a day to keep the fat away. I have been doing just that. I eat one apple after breakfast, one apple after lunch and one apple after dinner. It seems to be working.

Furthermore, my confidence has increased and I know that I can be victorious on my fight with M.S. I know that I can win and I am in the best shape of my life. My muscle mass has increased and I only weigh 180lbs. Not just that but my symptoms are under control. I no longer feel my face numb nor have I felt my tongue tangled up. There are still times when my jaw feels limited but it is not an everyday thing. I still have the spasms but it doesn't happen as often as it used too. I am jogging and my life feels great. This man knows what he is talking about and I know that if I keep doing what I am doing I will be cured.

The Truth

The truth is that even though most things seem to be in my favor, I am not happy with myself. I keep telling myself that I am but the truth is that I am not. I believe that if I can believe that I am happy then I will be happy. Unfortunately, the truth is that I have not yet find the success to be completely happy. Sure I got my symptoms under control, the tremors have stopped and I am in the best shape of my life. Not only am I down to 170 lbs, but I have started jogging, one thing that I never saw possible. The truth is that I feel trapped in a worthless body.

I am my own boss and I love it but the truth is that my sight is preventing me from becoming all that I can be. Primerica is a great business that allows me the opportunity to grow and get great compensation. Primerica has a lot of forms but frankly I have problems seeing these forms making it very difficult for me to complete them. The truth is that I rely on transportation to see my clients and with my sight the way it is I am a danger on the road. I have driven through several red lights and have had several close encounters. After avoiding several accidents on December 1, 2005 I was in an accident. My car is totaled but the good thing is that I am okay and nobody was hurt. Fearing for the life of other I decided to stop driving. I realized that life is too short and I don't want my journey to end with out me leaving my mark

I have gone to the optometrist several times now, but unfortunately they have not been able to help. They tell me that my eye sight changes to often and frankly the prescription would not help me. I may be a blinded man but I will still make a name for myself. M.S has not been able to stop me yet and I am not going to let this problem slow me down. I will figure it out even if I have to memorize every single form. I am frustrated that I cannot do a lot of things but I know that there will come a time when my frustration will be my salvation.

This is just another bump on the road and I will find a way around it. This bump will not stop me from driving in the flat road again.

Lost

Even though, I seem to be improving gradually I feel like everything is out of place in my life. It feels like nothing seems to be going my way. I don't know if I am walking forward or backwards anymore. I don't know if I am living days or just the same day over and over. I feel disoriented. I feel like there is nothing I can do to get out of this cycle. My heart is crying. I wish no more tears would fall. Love is too cruel and it doesn't allow me to forget. The memories I carry seem to take over my mind sometimes. I miss her. I feel alone and really need to forget. I am lost but I know I will find the right path again. I know this feeling won't last forever. How long I'll be lost who knows? But it won't be forever.

I feel lost and out of place. I should not be driving, but I do because it is a necessity. I know I put people's life in danger but my urge to survive on my own is stronger. I feel frustrated because I want to be something in life and my disabilities are stopping me from doing that. I want to help my parents, they mean the world. They are hard workers with low paying jobs and I don't want them working themselves to death. I want to supply them with enough income to make them retire and most importantly to get them out of their hard jobs. I want to help them so much but my disabilities are slowing me down. I guess that is why I take chances and the risk of driving to see clients. I am tired of not helping my parents. The reality is that I am a handicap but I just cannot accept that. I am a bit shaken up but I will not give into this feeling. I feel like I have lost my place in life. I hate this feeling. I hate not knowing what to do or where to go. I guess this is what they mean when people say "live life one day at a time". It is hard enough admitting that I am lost.

I find myself walking an empty dark road. I have no idea where I am walking to but I do know that I will not give up. I will find the right way home. I can't stop now. I must go on because my parents need me and I will not let them down. Life is a destiny I control. I know

I will find the right path. I will find a way to deal with my disabilities. I will survive. I will not let this dark road tell me where to go.

Death

Few people have heard my story. Those who have heard it tell me that I should become a motivational speaker. They have even told me that I am an inspiration in their life. Most of the times they still cannot believe that I have M.S. I guess it is because I do my best not to show my weaknesses. I may be an inspiration to people but I only see myself as an individual trying to survive.

Death is not something we look forward to, but we have no way of knowing when our time will expire. They say tomorrow never comes and I truly believe that is the truth. In my case I feel spiritually ready to go. If death comes knocking at my door I am willing to walk into its arms. There was a dark time when my depression was so deep that I asked never to wake up. Death was my only salvation. Fortunately, I kept waking up and I learned that life is precious and death is only a fear. A fear we should not be afraid to encounter.

The problems I have faced have made me wish I was dead so many times. Death seems to be the problem solver to most of my problems but somehow just by believing that I can do something I have managed to keep walking.

I think that my destiny has not been fulfilled yet and that is why I still walk among the living. I have been in several car accidents; accidents that have been my fault. My car has been completely totaled at times and yet I manage to escape with out a scratch. Maybe I am here to tell everyone my story. To share with everyone what I have found and to let everyone know my message. "It is not impossible to reach the untouchable." We just need to believe and not give up. We need to have faith in ourselves.

A New Start

As 2006 starts I begin the year without my car. My recent car accident has really made me think of not driving again. It is going to be extremely difficult but I have to try. My job depends on it and I am not sure I can stay away from the road. Not having my car is like asking an eagle to fly without its wings. I need my car. I need my freedom. I need to put an end to my loneliness and most importantly an end to my frustration.

This New Year will bring new opportunities, and new challenges that I will not back away from. Car or no car; I will not allow that to stop me. One of those opportunities has been the opportunity to expand my business. Unfortunately, I was unable to successfully pass my NASD licensing test due to me not being able to focus on the computer. You see I have to take this test at a testing center. There is also a time limit involved and frankly by the time my sight adapted to my surroundings it was to late. I needed to have passed the exam with a 70%. I scored a 65%. For a semi-blind person I did fairly well but I do not worry about it because I know this opportunity will cross roads with me again.

Multiple sclerosis is only a bump that will not stop me from making a name for myself. Memories will not slow me down. I breathe my destiny and have nothing to hide. I will see a better tomorrow. Multiple sclerosis may be a daily battle but I understand that it is not about wining the battles but the war.

I start 2006 with my symptoms under control. I continue to attend acupuncture and keep a strict diet. My body has not consumed any drug for almost three months now and I feel great. Dr. Skinner disapproves of my choice of not taking any drug. I look at myself and tell her that I am in the best shape of my life and that I now enjoy jogging every morning. I told her that I never felt that way while on the drugs. Exercise and a balanced diet are keeping me in control.

My sight has not improved and as long as I adapt to my surroundings I am okay. However, my numbness has decreased making movement easier. I am stronger than before and the hypersensitivity is more bearable than ever before. I can jog; something that appeared to be only a dream. My balance is almost normal and I no longer conceder tremors to be a big problem. The only thing that is really bothering me is that I am having problems opening my mouth. Multiple sclerosis is known for deforming the faces of other fighters. It is becoming very uncomfortable because there are times when I need to take a bite or yawn and I forget about my jaw and suddenly I am in pain because I tried to open my mouth more than its new limit. I have to take the time to find the spot where my jaw can open normally. It doesn't happen that often but I am still worried; so worried that I have start exercising my jaw by moving it around. Other than that I am happy with the fact that I am wining the war.

Early in the year I faced my first challenge. The flue took me out of commission. My eyes were so hypersensitive that it hurt to have them open. I felt so weak that I could hardly stand on my own two feet. My muscles ached and my body became number than usual. I feared that the flue would give M.S the opportunity to take control. It took a lot of rest, but after two weeks I am back in control.

Today is March 15, 2006; my 23rd birthday is only days away. A reminder of what has happened so far in my journey. I do not like making a big deal because for me it is just another day. A day that only brings back painful memories, and thoughts of what could have been. I will have dinner with the family, like very year, but for now I sit here on this cold night staring up into the stars. I sit here motionless under this dancing tree wishing I was cured. Alone, just me and my soul, thinking of what tomorrow may bring.

I know 2006 will be difficult. That is why I make no promises, but I hope that my loneliness comes to an end. I hope tomorrow will open windows of opportunities and that my business finally takes off.

My journey in life will go on, and I hope to leave my mark behind.

My Religion

Like you know I am not a religious person. I grew up in a catholic family but I really stopped believing in church at an early age. Faith is important no argument there, but some people really do not know what to believe in. People believe in a higher power and pray, asking the lord for forgiveness and to bring them joy. You're probably asking if I believe in God and to be honest with you I am not sure of the answer. Is there a God? Maybe I do not know. Is there a higher power? I think so. I think that there is a spirit in all of us that makes us who we are. It shows us the road; we just need to trust it. I know that the spirit within me has not allowed me to give up. I have taught of giving in so many times but somehow I never do.

My faith is in myself. I believe that if I can do something I will do it. If I want happiness I will get happiness simply by doing everything in my power to be happy. Right now for example. I am happy with myself because I have worked hard for it. I have kept a strict diet. I have exercise day in and day out and I feel great with my body. I feel free and if death knocks on my door I am ready to walk into its arms.

There is always a controversial discussion about what religion is the right one. The one religion that will take us to heaven. However, the truth is that there is no correct answer. Haven't you ever think that life is a test; a test to see who is worthy of even a better gift than life. We all know that complete happiness is only a dream that we all want. People pray and ask the lord to give them a space in his heaven, but what if there is no heaven. Why can't we be happy here? The truth is that we can. Nature has given us a great gift....our mind. No one person is alike and we all have the power to believe what ever we want. We are all different. I for example carry a unique signature. My palm prints are really something amazing. You see, when I put my palms next to each other, there is a straight line across my hands. It is a unique print that no one else in this entire world carries.

I carry a distinct mark and one of the most interesting disorders in this planet. What makes it even more amazing is that I was diagnosed at one of the earliest ages known to man. Don't tell me it is coincidence. It is destiny. I have faith in myself not in a god, and look at what I have accomplished. I have found no cure but I am happy with my life and with myself. I feel free.

Religion is the key to finding true happiness. Religion can do anything because it makes us believe that anything can happen. So, you see if we can think it, we can do it. We think with our minds and our mind is the most powerful of all gods. If we can believe it we can do it. If we can think it, it can happen. If we believe that we are happy we will be happy.

My religion is myself and my god is my mind. Because I can believe what I want I can do anything.

My religion is my cure and the way to true happiness.

My Final Message

I can't say that my life has been horrible because I know there are people out there that have it worse than me. However I will say that although my journey in life has been a short one, I have learned many lessons. I have learned that the most important lesson is to never give up because the odds can turn at any time. I have learned that sometimes all we have is faith and we have to hope for the best. Even though my struggles with multiple sclerosis continue I have adapted to my limits. I know that I will keep on fighting until I am cured. I understand that it may take my entire life but I have hope. Hope that multiple sclerosis is only a bump on the road that will not be able to stop me.

Multiple sclerosis is a very strange disorder and whether you're fighting MS or any other illness the cure is to never give up. Believe in yourself and in your dreams. Keep in mind that it is all mental. If we can believe that we can do it, we can do anything. Keep in mind that it is not impossible to reach the untouchable.

A Piece of My Mind

A piece of my mind is some of the things that I have written while relaxing at the beach or at the park. A piece of my mind is a way of expressing my feelings. I wrote these so called poems at different stages of my life; some while I was upset or mad, and wrote others while I was happy. I really do not think a piece of my mind as poetry but as thoughts. A piece of my mind is a way to forget about my fight with multiple sclerosis and I find writing to be very helpful. Sometimes a good cry makes everything better. A piece of my mind is me crying out to the world hoping that nobody is listening.

My Tragedy

July 20th, 2002   4 o'clock
My darkest hour
It only took a few words
Just like that dreams were shattered
My future disappeared
Pain like no other
Unimaginable…it hurts…it burns
Then I meat her
It hurt no more
A friend like no other
She promised never to leave
But she did
Waited impatiently but she never returned
It wasn't meant to be
I called and said goodbye one last time
My heart did not shatter
Overwhelmed by fire….pain gathered
I stand alone…fearing tomorrow
My memories….my yesterday
My tragedy

Obstacles

Life has been very hard for me
I've had so many obstacles
Yet I stand here on my own two feet looking
at everything that has happen
I have overcome everything that has stand
in my way
I will survive
With fear in my eyes I stand here...
ready to fight
Ready to overcome what ever is thrown
at me next
Nothing will stop me...I will go on
I have come so far that there is no point in
turning back....
I will survive....no obstacle can hold me back

Life

Sometime hard
Sometimes impossible
Sometimes understandable
Sometimes we want to give up
We just need to look back and remember
Sometimes we just have to push back
Life
If everything goes bad
Why push back
Life is unpredictable
The odds can flip at any time
We will have control
Love, happiness, laughter
Power, pain, and suffering
All in our hands
Life…we shouldn't give up
Don't make it stop
Life

Supernatural

It never ends…does it?
We go back an forth
You can't win…I won't let you
You're supernatural
You come out of no where
like lightning
You control my sight
my strength…my life
I've been blind
I've been down and out
Yet here I stand
Fighting this battle
Knowing the war is what matters

Time

I just can't tell anymore
Hours feel like minutes and days like hours
I don't know if I am living new days
Or just living the same day over and
over again
Time….the measurement of existence
Is traveling to fast to enjoy
Is it running out?….will it slow down?
Who knows…we shouldn't waste it looking
at yesterday
Let's just hope tomorrow does come
Time…..forgives no one
Let's not live the same day over and over
Leave the past in the past
Live today and hope for tomorrow

Death

A day with no sunshine
A night with no stars
The beginning or the end
Our final destination
Dark, quiet and peaceful
No time to prepare
Sometimes unpredictable
Sometimes unavoidable
Our time to rest
No more pain
No more worries
No more suffering
Death…the stairway to heaven
Happiness…and a better tomorrow
Death

To Be or Not To Be

I think the question should be
"Do you want it or not?"
If you want to be something
You first must aim at something
Sometimes it's easy
If you aim at nothing you're
guaranteed success
To be or not to be?
Be something...go get it
Be what you want to be
Do what you want to do
Become what you really want to be
To be or not to be...you decide
Take a stand

My Life

Life is a roller-coaster from hell
Life is hard but we don't want it to stop
Sometimes life is painful…cruel
Life is an endless road
Too many turns…and bumps on the road
Life is heaven
Life is a risky game
Take a chance…make every turn
It is unpredictable
unimaginable
Sometimes death is not an option
Life is an instinct
my life is difficult but it is also my heaven
my life is what I want it to be
my life…..my hell and my heaven
My life

Darkness

Inside I carry so many memories
Your words...your kisses...your touch
I fear this loneliness....this darkness
Your unreachable.....in other arms
I am desperate trying to reach you
Your silence imprisons me
Unreachable....lost in other arms
Unreachable....oh how I hurt inside
Just to hold you one more time
Darkness

Who I Am

I am not who I appear to be
My actions define who I really am
I am not about diamonds, rubies or emeralds
I am not about wasting time
I am about life and it doesn't stop
I am about happiness
About having clean fun
I am about following my heart
About using my head
About not giving up
I am a fighter......I am a survivor
I am about leaving my mark in time
I know that it is not about winning the battle
But winning the war
I am a dreamer with big dreams
A romantic without words
I am a man with a big heart
My actions define who I am

Love

Love is blind and unexpected
Love is like a miracle…it's hard to explain
Love is when you feel complete
Love is thinking with your heart not
your head
Love is the wish of holding you
the fear of loosing you
the anxiety to be with you
Love is when I close my eyes and
only see you
Love is saying "I am sorry" when we fight
Love is suffering when you're gone
Love is happiness
the peacefulness when I hold you
Love is the great feeling when I hear
your voice

Love is when I dream awake
Love is when you're the only thing I can
think of
Love is a beautiful thing
But if we are not careful it makes life
miserable
It becomes our worst enemy
It is cruel and forgives no one
Love hurts....love scares
Love is like a flame....
It burns when it's hot
Love is a force not to be wrecked with
Sometimes it is only a desire...a wish
Sometimes only a dream

Thinking of You

You make me go crazy
I think of you every second
I see you everywhere
At the store…work…in my car
You're every where
Insanely in love
Desperate for your touch
Your smile…your laugh…your eyes
I want to run my fingers thru your hair
hold you in my arms
I need the sweetness in your lips
the brightness in your eyes
Thinking of you

One Last Time

The sky is red
like when you blush
The sky and the sea are one
it's like looking into your eyes
The air is clean
fresh like your scent
The city is a ghost town
Time doesn't move
I want to see you
hear your whispers
Kiss you like yesterday
Let's live
be my princess
The night is cold
like your goodbye
Keep me warm
one last time

You

Frighten of tomorrow
Scared of the world
Love may be blinding
You own my eyes and my soul
The waves are strong
the nights are cold
The stars don't glow
I cry inside when you're gone
I am falling for you
Always thinking of you
You said you would call
I live by the phone…desperately waiting
your call
I didn't think this would happen
I'm falling desperately for you
I wasn't expecting it
I love you more everyday
Falling for you

How Dare You

How dare you call
when you know I'm with someone
Someone who picked up the pieces of my
broken heart
Someone who put an end
to my misery…my loneliness
How dare you call after hurting me
You know I'm with someone
The one person who has healed
the scar you left behind
How dare you

Sometimes

Sometimes you're pretty cute
Sometimes you're crazy beautiful
Sometimes we need to slow down and
smell the roses
Sometimes what we want is right under
our noses
Sometimes we need to explore
we need to take a chance
Sometimes we think things through
Sometimes we just follow our heart
Sometimes we want to talk
Sometimes we need to listen
Sometimes all we need is a smile
Sometimes a smile makes everything better
Sometimes we just want to be a kid
hope for a miracle

Sometimes we need someone to care
Someone to talk to
Someone to listen
Someone to laugh with
Someone to smile back
Sometimes a giggle is good for the soul
Sometimes an aching soul needs a cure
Sometimes love is the cure
love is the answer
Sometimes love is risky
Sometimes the heart doesn't care
Sometimes.....all it takes is a phone call
Sometimes
all it takes is you

When?

When was the last time you saw the stars
with your eyes closed
When was the last time you dreamed awake
when?
When was the last time you touched the stars
When was the last time a simple déjà vu
became more
When was the last time love left because it
wanted to be free
When?
When was the last time you let the spark
in your heart burn
When was the last time you touched the stars
the last time silence became a melody
When was the last time a simple déjà vu
became more
When?
When was the last time you walked on air
the last time you took a chance at love
When?

I Need

Someone to inspire me
Who will push me harder than anyone else
Someone to talk to....someone to listen
Someone to make laugh when she cries
Someone to tell I love you
I will walk until I find her
Someone to end my loneliness
Someone to fill this emptiness in my heart
Someone to make laugh when she cries
Someone to smile back
Are you what I need?
I need someone to care
Someone to laugh with me
Someone to enjoy life with
Someone to make laugh when she cries
I need...to find you

Maybe

Maybe time doesn't want us together
Maybe life hides the truth from us
Maybe because of life I search non stop
I know deep inside we are one
You never know if tomorrow will come
I go crazy….just knowing you're out there
Maybe our roads won't cross
Maybe you walk towards the moon
While I walk towards the sun
I know deep inside we are one hot flame
And belong together
Maybe time is running out
Maybe we will never find each other
Who knows…maybe you're a dream
an illusion
Maybe time will keep us apart
Maybe I will never find you
I know I won't stop until I have you
Maybe

Desperate

Desperate for the day
When everything is normal
Desperate to get out
for an exit…the solution
No way out…I am trapped
Desperate for air…for freedom
The walls are falling in
I must get out
Desperate for the answer to my prayers
for the impossible
For a way out
Desperate for a cure

Tired

Tired of walking alone
Tired of walking in the dark
Too tired to go on.....just too tired
Tired of life...of playing this game
Tired of caring this darkness....this emptiness
this pain in my soul.... I am tired
My reason to give up
Tired of things not going my way
Too tired to go on
Tired of this lonely road
of not finding you
It's heavy...just too heavy
The pain in my soul is too heavy
I am tired

My Frustration

Tired of not being able to do anything
Tired of needing help
Frustrated of wanting to do more and not
being able too
of not being able to help
Tired of others always looking over me
Frustrated of not being like the past
Frustrated of not being all that I can be
Tired of needing help
Frustrated of living in the present
When I want my past
Tired of waiting
My frustration

Lost

I am out of place
Time is running by to fast
Leaving me disoriented
I don't know if I am walking forward
or backwards
I don't know where I am headed
Lost in transition…not knowing where to go
Am I walking through the past or
to the future
The present doesn't feel right
Lost….frustrated…confused and disoriented
Out of place and time is running out
I just don't know what way to walk anymore
The world is spinning and there is nothing
to grab on to
Time is playing with me
I don't know where to go
Lost in transition…not knowing where to go

Promise Me

If you promise to come back
If you promise to return
With my eyes closed I wait
I will count the cold and windy nights
without you
promise to come back
When I hold you I discover the stars
The earth rumbles and silence becomes
a melody
I resuscitate with your touch
For good or worse...I will be here
Your love will never die....even if you
need to depart
Time will not keep us apart
If you promise to come back
Come back soon...I need you

This stormy night scares me
When I'm with you there is no fear…
no shadows
I need you
I need the music of your happiness
The hours taste better when I am
in your arms
I will wait
I will count the nights without you
for every night I will fall in love
with you again
I need you….I am nothing without you
Please promise to come back

My Nightmare

One more day with out you
I only think of you
Life seems impossible
Here is my heart do what ever you want
my soul is waiting for you
Here is my blood that still runs fast when I
hear of you
Here are my dreams and my future
You're cruel but I need you
Here is my body...do what you want of it
Here is my soul the only thing you
can't break
Take my heart that still beats harder
when I hear you
Rip it out from my chest
Here is the end to my dreams
my desires
One more day without you
You left my arms at sunrise
you said no goodbye
It's a nightmare

Let Me Be

Everything I got I owe to you
I wait for the wind to blow in my favor
So many memories between you and me
Who would have though of you leaving
my side
I only live for you
So many promises that have turn into
endless dreams
I need you....nothing seems impossible
with you
Even my tears miss you
So many moments...I insist
Leaving was a mistake
Since I laid eyes on you...I only live for you
I know you're not only for me
Just let me be

Straight to the Heart

I can't take another lie
You won't fool me
No second chance….no do over
I know it hurts….don't be afraid
don't look back
Try not to shake
Just stab….straight to the heart
Please not in the back
Just shoot…straight to the heart
Look me in the eyes
Blind fold me if you like
pull, squeeze and shoot
I am already dead….just shoot
Straight to the heart

Thoughts

Two times the trouble
different consequences
A good and a bad
maybe just a bad
Too many ideas
Can't make it stop
Love it or hate it
a good and a bad
Sweet or bitter…happy or sad
Always in my mind
Thoughts

Endless Night

One, two, three, four…ten
Wish I was counting money
I would be a millionaire
Can't sleep…so I think
I listen to the whispers of the night
I stare into its dark eyes
Can't see it's to dark
I'm going insane
Minutes feels like hours
Hours like days
An endless night

A Pain Within

Don't cry for me
Tears won't bring us back
Let it be....I don't want to see you cry
Your tears make me suffer
I can't lie....and it's hard to hide what you
make me feel
You're my world...my destiny...my future
Let it be......don't cry
What we have is special
It's hard to find...it doesn't come and go
Time travels slowly when I hold you
I need you
I would do anything to be with you
I would bring you the stars
make the impossible possible
I would cross land and sea...just to hold you

You're everything that matters
My tears will make an ocean if you leave
I will swim non stop
Just to see you one more time
If you leave....pain will eat me alive
my heart will burn
I won't last a day without you
There is so much love
But time says..."it's time to go"
Let it be....set me free

One More Drink

To get rid of her taste
To wash away the pain she left
I loved you like no other
like no one else can...you meant the world
Life is tough
Your life is not a carnival
you don't come and go
One more bottle
To wash away my memories
my anger...my life
Stay...don't leave
Keep me from drowning
Safe me...don't walk away
Bartender..."one more drink"

Today

Today for the first time I realized that
there is only one like you
I know...I left without saying goodbye
But with every step I take I am
reminded of you
Today I see myself in the mirror
And only see emptiness
I see pain that has left a big scar
I will return
I am not the same and I need you
I will return because I drown without you
There is only one like you
I miss you
Today I realized the scar can heal
I will return...because I know you
wait for me
I will return because I need you
I will return....because that is
what the heart wants
Today I realized that there is
only one like you
Just one....and I want you

Mistakes

Look at me when I tell you I love you
Kiss me like the first time
Hug me and don't let go
Let yourself go with your emotions
it's okay to be angry…to cry
Maybe it's too late to beg
Give me a second chance
Look at me…when I tell you that I love you
Hug me and don't let me free
I promise to be there when the sun rises
Maybe it is too late
Maybe I should not get that chance
I am miserable…look at me

Fly Back

Come back
don't go
Wake me with your whispers
With your singing
Heaven calls
Don't leave.....come back
My ears bleed without you
I need you
your singing...your voice
Don't leave
Fly back

Alone

I walk alone
This empty....dark road
No sun...no moon....no stars
I am scare....hold my hand
Don't know where this road goes
I walk alone.....this empty road
Alone...not knowing where I go
Nothing to my left...nothing to my right
And definitely nothing in front
I walk alone...this empty road
Alone just me and my soul
Alone...not knowing where to go
Alone

My Emptiness

I am nothing without you
Everything I do is because of you
Everything I have…you've given to me
All your words are of love
my desires are of you
You're my past, present and future
I only see your light
Nothing else matters
Without you I am lost
All my memories are of you
My only illusion is to see you laugh
I only want to stand by you
Now that you're no longer here
The silence of the night kills me
This emptiness
only you can fill

Live or Die

Maybe you have not realized that you and I
are not like yesterday
Maybe your scare…maybe your scare to let go
May be you fear not seeing me again
Maybe you fear I will change
you think I will stop loving you
there is life ahead
Maybe you think life will make me forget
Maybe things between us will change
Maybe I'll live
Maybe I'll die
But in your arms I will end up
Live or die
I will wait for you in the end
Live or die in your arms I will end up

I Breathe

I breathe my destiny
I know what is to come
I stare into the sunset with nothing to hide
Someday the shadows will be the light
the stars will no longer be bright
Someday the roads will cross
I'll just follow the hiding lights
Someday I will be out of breath
But till then not you nor God
Can tell me what to breathe
I breathe my destiny
And follow my dreams

Freedom

My desire
A dream difficult to follow
No stress…no worries…..
no hesitation…..freedom
Just to be able to open my wings
and be able to fly away
Sore through the sky and be free
like no other
Freedom
To fear nothing and roar like no other
To stretch my legs and run as fast as I want
To conquer anything that stands in my way
But yet be peaceful and beautiful
Like a butterfly flying from lily to lily
Freedom…..my dream….my desire

Friends

Good friends are hard to find
But I am as good as they come
If they need to talk…. I listen
If they need help…..I help
If they have a problem….I solve it
A good friend
But when the roles are reversed
Their backs are turned
I need new friends
But why have them
You know what they say
Keep your friends close and
Your enemies closer
Friends

Story of My Life

July 20, 2002 a new beginning
An unexpected change
A turn for the worst
Just like that I was screwed
My back is against the wall
So weak…can't walk and can't see
wish I would just die
I am no looser…I couldn't just give up
I am in the dark….alone and scared
Yet I survived…once again…the odds are
in my favor
Battle after battle…I am winning
I must be careful
One move away from being screwed…
Suddenly….a big bang
Just like that I was screwed
Life is hard…too unexpected…
too unpredictable
Just like that…I was in the dark
Game over….try again
The story of my life

It's All the Same

Live or die
It makes no difference…it doesn't matter
Dead or alive
You'll be gone…It's all the same
Your lies may fool me
But your eyes don't
Love or hate
it's all the same
This is no game
we could get hurt
Your love may fool me
But your eyes won't
live or die
It's all the same

Addiction

Addicted to survival
To freedom....to life
Addicted to the nectar in you
To your touch.....your lips
to the heaven in your eyes
Addicted to your smile...your laughter
Addicted to fighting.....to this darkness
To these memories....this life
this misery
Addicted to surviving
to you

Keep Me

I can only breathe with you
I can only reach the clouds with you
Don't take away my wings
Teach me to fly higher
to breathe in outer space
Keep me a live
Show me the future
Make time infinite
Stand by me
Keep me breathing
Show me how to breathe under water
Fly with me.....explore with me.....
cry with me
Be free with me....I die without you
Keep me...survive with me
Live life...keep me

My Necessity

A window of opportunity
A chance to redeem myself
I need to prove...I am worth it
I need to explore...I need to get out
I need your inspiration...your smile...
your laughter
I need you like the ocean needs salt
like the air I breathe
I need you....my soul mate...my confident
I need to take a chance
I need to hope for the best
Get me out of my misery
Help me out
I need your strength...your support
Your love

Trapped

Singing birds outside my window
Trapped with no way out
In between four walls...running out of air
Trapped in this hell hole
No way out...trapped
Trapped in a worthless body
Running out of air
Roses grow outside my window
Trapped without their scent
Trapped....no way out
I am going crazy....I must get out
Trapped in my body
Trapped...no way out

Scared

Scared of sitting in this chair
Always being pushed around
Scared of sitting here watching life go by
without me
Scared of not being on my feet
Scared of fear….scared of this dark road
Scared of sitting here not able to do anything
of not being able to fly away
Scared of this emptiness
of the tears in the mirror
Scared of dieing without you
Hold me…..I'm scared

Face to Face

We met very young
I love you more than yesterday
Yet you hate me like no other
I am standing right here
don't run
You kick me when I am down
You control the odds
Yet I continue on my feet
running into your arms
You may be wining the battle
but the war is mine
I am scared to death
I shake in my boots....cry in the dark
See me in the eyes...look at me
I am not giving up
With fear in my eyes...I stand
Face to face....eye to eye
Kill me if you dare....but it won't
put me down
Take your best shot.....I'll get up
Face to face...eye to eye...we stand

One Day

Just one day of normality
One day when I can play ball
One day to keep my hope alive
Just one day to make new memories
just one day
One day to feel your face…..your hair
One day to be free
A day to be normal
Just one day with no pain…no loneliness
No darkness….one day to dream awake
One day to run in the rain
one day

White Rose

Soft…elegant…sincere
Pure…and beautiful
You just want to stand out
Let your beauty roar…capture the world
You scent conquers the winds
your beauty my eyes
Soft…elegant…beautiful
Can't look away
Your light grows in my heart
The soil for your beauty
The one place you will always live in
Soft…elegant….and beautiful

Angel Eyes

The sunshine to my heart
the window to heaven
The sun in your eyes
So sweet…so breath taking
those eyes
Brighter than the stars
You light up my nights
my life…my heart
those eyes
The door to heaven
to peace…to happiness
Angel eyes

Know Me

You still don't know me
Love runs inside
Hug me…kiss me…love me
This time just with your eyes
Let yourself go….lets live
You still don't know me
Slow down….look at me
Undress me….with your eyes
Don't turn this into an adventure
You still don't know me

Just My Imagination

If I could only be with you
Holding you in my arms
staring at you in the silence
Just to have you in my arms
If I could only tell you how you make me feel
Just to have you here
To be able to stare into your eyes and
see the stars
We can stare at the moon....fly like light flies
Let one more day go by
Just to be able to think you're crazy about me
If I could only be with you
keep you warm when night falls
Just to have you in my arms
Just my imagination

When Night Falls

Kiss me goodnight…..hold me
One final goodbye
I welcome yesterday
Overwhelmed by darkness
I shut my eyes…and think
The stars shine…the moon glows
heaven smiles
It is cool…he wind whispers
When night falls
Let me hold you…I'll keep you warm
Shut your eyes and think
The stars shine…the moon glows
heaven smiles
When night falls

You and I

It will always be you....I need nothing more
When I look at you I feel in space
You will always be my dream
my desire....my love....my life
We will reach the stars
The air doesn't taste the same without you
I can't breathe
You will always be my everything
my life...my passion
Nothing can keep us apart
You and I

Beside Your Bed

Waking to my scent…my breath
my presence
Waking with a sparkle on your eyes
seeing me in the far
The smile on my face…your taste on my lips
Remember yesterday
What we shared…the time we spent
The memories we created
that now sit on this vase
Beside your bed
the rose I gave you rests

Like I Do

Who's going to love you
Who will kiss you good night
Who will cry your tears
Who will laugh your laughter
like I do
Who will talk....listen to you
Who will cry your tears
laugh your laughter
love you
Like I do

Against all Odds

Just want to find you
I'll face anything in my way
Lightning…thunder….the impossible
Just to be with you
No fear of what may come
Just want to hold you
The past was yesterday
The future starts today
I'll face the odds
the winds….the rain…the gods…
the impossible
Not scared of anything
live or die
Against all odds….just to be with you

Loving You

I fall for you
and you don't see me
You're in my head
in my dreams…my days…my nights
Spring is in the air
Your scent in the wind
Romance in my vanes
I fall for you
I go crazy thinking of you
Desperately awaiting a sign
Love is in the air
With my eyes closed
I'm falling for…you

I Like You

I like your eyes....you mouth
your lips...your smile
Your present...your yesterday
I like everything
I like your touch....your hands
your soul....I like you
I like to wake up thinking
I'm going to see her
Thinking you like me
I like the way you make me feel
How you make the butterflies
in my tummy roar
I like your face...your eyes
you smile...your laugh
I like you

One Kiss

Just one...that's all it takes
To walk on air...to touch the moon
I'll bring you a star
That's all it takes to turn me crazy
Just to taste the nectar in your lips
the honey in you smile
One kiss...to fall in love
Just one...to dream awake
Just one....to walk on air
One kiss....to love you
to find paradise
One kiss

Sunrise

You come thru my window
you kiss me good morning
My nightmare begins
Time to go for a jog
too weak to get up
Can't feel my feet
can't see...I'm blind
No feeling in my hands
too weak to get up
Must get up...the sun is up
Time to go to war
Its sunrise

Sunshine

You bring the warmth
to my life…to my heart
The light…the brightness
You show me the way
what road to follow
You light up my heart
my destiny…my dreams
Your kiss in the morning
Your honeydew eyes staring down on me
Staring thru my window
Good morning, sunshine

My Confident

You're always there…thank you
So comforting…so soft
Ready to listen…ready to help
You've seen me cry…you've seen me smile
Yet you tell no one…thank you
You're always there….to listen
to wipe my tears
A friend like no other
as helpful as can be
No matter how late it may be…you're there
Holding my head…filling the emptiness
in my bed
Keeping me company…always by me
My best friend…my confident
Thanks

Sadness

The past is nothing more
Sad of the memories
The heart just can't forget
Sad of being trapped in the past
The pain won't go away
An apology is not enough
The heart doesn't forget
Memories can't be erased
Sad of what happened….sad of my life
Sad of the actions
but once done…their done
Sad

My Suffering

Trapped
Between what's real and what's not
I can't deny it…you're forbidden
Yesterday still hurts
Suffering from something that may not exist
I'm dieing…I can't breathe
The air isn't the same
Trapped…no way out
Nights are painful and empty
Yesterday still hurts
Trapped…between what's real and what's not
Suffering…no way out

Frighten

Frighten of seeing the minutes go by
with out you
Frighten of not being able to hold you
Frighten of this loneliness in space
of the face in the mirror
Frighten of this fear
of this illness
Frighten of saying goodbye
Of not feeling your face...of seeing your
sad eyes
Frighten of seeing you cry
Frighten...of never seeing you again
Frighten

Reality

The truth is painful
Yesterday never leaves
Tomorrow never comes
Nothing goes my way
My back is against the wall
reality
I will never find you
The war is eternal
Life hurts…it's too lonely
Hope is my salvation
Days are miserable
Nights are desperate
Reality

My Passion

Nothing will stop me
I'll be your star from above
I'll become stronger than this earth
Nothing will stop me
I will run to you…dream of you
Watch over you
You may be a dream but you're not
unreachable
Nothing will stop me
I will survive
I will bring you the stars
My passion

The Day

When the day comes…I'll know
The sun won't shine
the stars won't glow
Birds won't sing…flies won't fly
the rain won't stop
Darkness will fall
That's how I'll know
The war will stop
A winner will be crowned
time to go home
The day I die
hope never comes

Fantasy

I dream of the day
when life is simple
Of the eyes
I've never seen
I dream awake or asleep
day or night
Under the sun or the stars
Of the happiness I need
Of your face
something I've never seen
I dream of you lips
a flavor I haven't taste
Of the kiss that never happened
I dream

If I Only Had One Wish

Just one wish….that's all I ask for
to save me from this nightmare
One chance to change
to start over
One inspiration to keep me going
One wish….one miracle
One wish to end this dream….this illusion
This nightmare
One wish to start over.
Just one chance
If I only had one wish

Silent Whispers

Yesterday is calling
a voice that never stays in the past
It never leaves
It haunts us
always ringing in our ears
always in our head
and only we can hear
it is the voice of yesterday's spirit
calling out our actions
preparing us for tomorrow
Silent Whispers

The Window

we all look at it different
for some it is an opportunity
for others a waste of time
yet it is the same thing
sometimes we like what we see
sometimes we get scare
we can run away from it
yet it always embraces us
it is something to hate
to fear, to cherish…to love
just open the window

As I Wait

the day is near
only hours away
but I seat here
looking into the eyes of yesterday
wondering about tomorrow
hoping for better opportunities
in the mirror I see
the face of the monster I've become
Life has been cruel
unpredictable and unexpected
the road to success was altered
I am lost trying to find the right path
as I wait the day when it all changes
the day to celebrate a new beginning
the day to forget about yesterday
As I wait

Fantasy

I dream of the day
when life is simple
Of the eyes
I've never seen
I dream awake or asleep
day or night
Under the sun or the stars
Of the happiness I need
Of the peace
only you can bring
Of your face
something I've never seen
I dream of you lips
a flavor I haven't taste
Of the kiss that never happened
I dream

Sleepless Night

One, two, three, four...ten
Wish I was counting money
I would be a millionaire
Can't sleep...so I think
I listen to the whispers of the night
I stare into its dark eyes
Can't see it's to dark
I'm going insane
Minutes feels like hours
Hours like days
An endless night

Supernatural

It never ends…does it?
We go back an forth
You can't win…I won't let you
You're supernatural
You come out of no where
like lightning
You control my sight
my strength…my life
I've been blind
I've been down and out
Yet here I stand
Fighting this battle
Knowing the war is what matters

Rain Falls

It's cold outside
the air is misty, cold
yet it whispers
the moon is no where
yet it shines
the sky is dark
chills run down my spine
the streets are quiet
birds hide…the trees dance
all the bad is gone
washed away…it won't be back
peace falls
when rain falls

978-0-595-39290-2
0-595-39290-3

www.ingramcontent.com/pod-product-compliance
Lightning Source LLC
Chambersburg PA
CBHW030257290526
45785CB00001B/123